CHOLESTEROL:
Questions You Have ... Answers You Need

CHOLESTEROL:

Questions You Have ... Answers You Need

Ellen Moyer

Consultant editor Dr Robert Youngson

Thorsons
An Imprint of HarperCollinsPublishers

Thorsons
An Imprint of HarperCollins*Publishers*
77–85 Fulham Palace Road,
Hammersmith, London W6 8JB
1160 Battery Street,
San Francisco, California 94111–1213
Published by Thorsons 1998

1 3 5 7 9 10 8 6 4 2

A catalogue record for this book
is available from the British Library

ISBN 0 7225 3543 0

Printed and bound in Great Britain by
Caledonian International Book Manufacturing Ltd, Glasgow

CONTENTS

PUBLISHER'S NOTE

INTRODUCTION

The relationship between blood cholesterol and health is far too important to be misunderstood. And, unfortunately, there are more misconceptions about this subject than about almost any other health issue. Regrettably, much of this misinformation is spread in books and articles written by people who have little real understanding of what is, in fact, a far more complex subject than most people appreciate. Moreover, the rate of progress of knowledge on the subject has recently been so great that nearly all the popular books already published on the matter are already seriously out of date.

This remarkably informative and reliable book explains, in a direct, simple and yet authoritative manner, all the important facts about cholesterol and its relationship to a disease that has been described as 'the number one killer of the Western world': atherosclerosis. In our pampered and overfed society, this arterial disease – intimately related to cholesterol – is responsible for more deaths and serious damage to the quality of life than any other single condition. It is the cause of heart attacks, angina pectoris, strokes, gangrene of the limbs, a form of severe kidney damage and other human disasters. A number of things promote this dangerous condition, but it is now established that one of the major risk factors is an undue rise in the level of certain cholesterol-carriers in the blood. So knowledge about cholesterol can be literally vital.

This book, the result of long and patient study by a dedicated student of the subject who has interviewed many notable experts and studied their professional papers, brings together in an easy-to-understand and readable question-and-answer format all the essential facts about cholesterol. This is a balanced account which illuminates facts that will surprise, and perhaps alarm, most readers. It does not hesitate to highlight those areas on which medical opinion is divided or about which the scientists have had to admit ignorance. But research has now provided us with a great deal of hard information about cholesterol – how it is formed, how it is transported, how it can aid us and how it can damage us. All this is clearly explained. The book covers the question of diet and cholesterol thoroughly, and explains the action and value of the range of drugs which can be used to control the forms of cholesterol-carriers which are, in excess, dangerous. The relationship of cholesterol to fats (triglycerides) is also clearly explained.

In short, this book tells you everything you need to know about an important subject, and how best to benefit from this knowledge in the interests of your own health and longevity. It is a book which could be of the first importance to you and it will repay your close attention.

Dr R. M. Youngson, Series Editor
London, 1998

CHAPTER ONE

CHOLESTEROL BASICS

Q   I know that having high **cholesterol** is supposed to be
     bad for me, and that cholesterol is somehow related to
     fat, but beyond that, I'm in the dark. So what exactly is
     cholesterol?

A   Cholesterol is a white, waxy substance found naturally
     throughout the body, including in the blood. It is essential
     for good health.

     Technically, cholesterol is not a fat but a closely
     related substance. It belongs to a class of compounds
     called **sterols**. But it is often called a blood fat, or **lipid**.

     Like any wax or fat, cholesterol does not dissolve in
     water. So in the blood, cholesterol is carried around in
     an envelope of protein. This cholesterol-protein package,
     called a **lipoprotein** (of which there are several kinds),
     does stay soluble in the watery serum portion of the
     blood.

     That's why, when doctors measure cholesterol, they
     often do it in two ways: first they measure total choles-
     terol – all the cholesterol in your blood. Then they
     measure each of the different lipoproteins in your blood

which, together, make up your total cholesterol. Each amount is measured as milligrams per decilitre (mg/dL). We'll explain more about these different lipoproteins later in this chapter.

Q **What about triglycerides? Aren't they related to cholesterol?**

A Not really. Triglycerides are also fats, or lipids, but they have a chemical structure that is different from cholesterol's. A triglyceride molecule contains three chains of fat – actually fatty acids – hence the 'tri' prefix. And instead of being attached to a protein molecule, they are attached to a glycerine (glycerol) molecule, which, like protein, is soluble in the watery serum part of the blood.

Q **Does a triglyceride molecule contain cholesterol?**

A No, it is a completely different fat.

Q **Where do cholesterol and triglycerides come from?**

A You can get both cholesterol and triglycerides from dietary sources – foods.

Cholesterol comes only from the animal foods you eat. Triglycerides are found in both animal fats and plant oils. Organ meats, such as liver and brains, contain lots of cholesterol, as do egg yolks, shrimp and lobster. Other meats, butter and whole milk also contain substantial amounts.

However, you may be surprised to learn that your liver actually makes about two-thirds of the cholesterol and some of the triglycerides in your body.

Q   How does the liver make cholesterol and triglycerides?

A   To make cholesterol, the liver uses the fats you eat, primarily **saturated fats**, such as butter or lard, which are solid at room temperature. That's one reason a high saturated-fat diet tends to lead to high blood-cholesterol levels. In the case of triglycerides, both alcohol and sugar increase the liver's production.

Q   What exactly does cholesterol do? You said earlier that it is essential for good health.

A   Cholesterol does serve a useful purpose. It is needed by the body to make hormones, including sex hormones and adrenal hormones, and to make vitamin D. It's also needed to produce bile acids, which aid fat absorption in the small intestine, and to build cells, especially the fatty membranes which enclose cells and the structures within cells.

Q   And what do triglycerides do?

A   They provide fats which are either burned for energy or deposited into the body's fat stores – the fat found under your skin and around your middle – to be used later for energy.

Q   It sounds like we need this stuff. Then why is having high cholesterol considered to be so bad?

A   High cholesterol, by itself, isn't a disease. It's simply a measurement that's used to assess your *risk* of disease. And certainly not everyone with high cholesterol develops health problems.

On the other hand, studies show that, in general, people with high blood levels of cholesterol are more likely than people with normal or low levels to develop a disease in which some of the cholesterol sticks to the inner surfaces of blood vessels, causing **atherosclerosis**. **Coronary artery disease** is the most common and serious result. We explain in Chapter 4 why having very low cholesterol might also be a problem for some people.

Q **Before we go on, what's considered a high blood level of cholesterol?**

A These days, most doctors consider any level over 200 mg/dL to be a potential problem, depending on other risk factors you may also have. And levels over 240 mg/dL definitely put you at higher risk of developing atherosclerosis.

Q **And what is coronary artery disease? Heart disease?**

A It's a specific kind of heart disease. Coronary artery disease is atherosclerosis of the coronary arteries, the spaghetti-sized arteries that deliver blood to the muscle of the heart.

Q **Atherosclerosis. Is that hardening of the arteries?**

A Well, almost. Atherosclerosis is a medical term which refers specifically to the gradual build-up of fatty deposits, called **plaque**, on the inside walls of the arteries.

A similar word, **arteriosclerosis**, literally means 'hardening of the arteries'. It is a broad term – now rather out of date – used to cover a variety of diseases, including atherosclerosis, which lead to abnormal thickening and hardening of the artery walls.

Q **But as for atherosclerosis – how does cholesterol end up on artery walls?**

A Only the cholesterol carried in the **low-density lipoproteins** (LDL for short) ends up on artery walls in any appreciable amounts. In studies, people with high levels of LDL have an increased risk of atherosclerosis. On the other hand, people with high amounts of another type of lipoprotein, **high-density lipoprotein** (HDL), have a reduced risk of atherosclerosis.

LDL CHOLESTEROL

Q **Is cholesterol in LDLs the kind that's called 'bad' cholesterol?**

A Yes. LDLs contain lots of cholesterol. Their job in the body is to transport cholesterol from the liver to the cells. If there is more cholesterol available than cells can take up and use, LDL ends up circulating in the bloodstream until, eventually, it gets deposited in artery walls.

Q **Does it accumulate just anywhere?**

A It tends to stick in places where the innermost layer of cells – a protective barrier of **endothelial cells** – has been damaged. It sticks to the walls of arteries which have microscopic tears or rough spots as a result of high blood pressure, toxin damage from cigarette smoke, or bacterial or viral infections, and in places where blood flow is turbulent because the artery branches or because circulation has been altered by bypass surgery.

Q   So that's all? It just piles up on artery walls and eventually blocks them off?

A   No, the process is fairly complicated, at least by microscopic standards. The LDL cholesterol, which is a relatively small molecule, squeezes through the spaces between the lining cells (endothelial cells) until it is inside the wall of the artery. There, it reacts with oxygen in a chemical process called **oxidation** (which, incidentally, certain vitamins can help to stop; we talk more about the protective role of **antioxidant** vitamins in Chapter 5).

Once the LDL cholesterol is oxidized, the process really takes off. The oxidized LDL tends to draw more LDL towards it, like a magnet. Then **macrophages**, immune-system scavenging cells designed to clean up messes, move in and gobble up the oxidized LDL cholesterol.

Q   So these cells clean up this mess?

A   No, in this particular situation they just seem to make it worse. If LDL levels remain high, macrophages seem to get too much of it and, literally, die of overeating the oxidized LDL. In the process they turn into **foam cells** — large, fluffy cells which, under a microscope, really do look foamy. The foam cells die, spilling their contents within the artery wall and causing cracks in the artery wall which attract **platelets** — small, disc-shaped structures involved in blood coagulation. These platelets secrete chemicals which attract smooth muscle cells. These grow, become degenerate and form scar tissue. Later, calcium in the bloodstream may cover the whole mess with a hard shell. This dangerous new mass is called an atherosclerotic plaque.

Q **So the plaque – which I thought was just a deposit of cholesterol in the artery – contains a lot of different things, not just cholesterol.**

A Yes. The plaque consists of cholesterol, other lipids, fibrous materials, cellular debris and minerals.

In fact, there are two different kinds of plaque. The one we've just described is called active plaque, and while it has the greatest potential for causing problems – because it's most likely to cause blood clots – it is also the only type which seems able actually to shrink in size, given the proper conditions. We talk about the regression of heart disease in Chapter 5.

The other type of plaque is mostly cholesterol encased in scar tissue. It may be older than active plaque and has no signs of macrophage activity. It usually doesn't cause problems, but it doesn't shrink, either.

Q **What's considered a good level of LDL to have?**

A Below 130 mg/dL is considered desirable. Borderline high is 130 to 159 mg/dL, and high is 150 mg/dL or above. People who have heart disease are advised to try to keep their LDL cholesterol levels at 100 mg/dL or lower.

TRIGLYCERIDES

Q **Do triglycerides build up on artery walls?**

A There is very little evidence that triglycerides build up, or deposit, on artery walls.

Q **But isn't a high blood level of triglycerides potentially harmful?**

A A high blood level of triglycerides, by itself, may not be so bad. But high triglyceride levels frequently go hand-in-hand with low levels of so-called 'good' HDL cholesterol (which we discuss in a minute) and often with high levels of LDL cholesterol.

One study, the Helsinki Heart Study, found that people with high blood triglyceride levels alone – no other risk factors – had about a 50 per cent increased risk of coronary artery disease, compared with people with normal levels.

However, they had a three-fold risk of coronary artery disease when they had both high blood triglyceride levels and low levels of HDL. And their risk for developing coronary artery disease was five times greater compared with people with desirable levels of triglycerides when they also had at least borderline high blood pressure (140/90 mmHg or above.) So it seems probable that triglycerides do most of their dirty work when other risk factors are present.

Further, recent studies suggest that high triglyceride levels make blood more readily form clots, another important factor in clogged arteries.

Q   **What is considered a high level of triglycerides?**

A   Levels above 500 mg/dL are considered very high, and 250 to 500 borderline high. For most people, levels below 200 are considered normal. We have more to say about ranges of triglycerides in Chapter 3.

HDL CHOLESTEROL

Q   **So now I know about 'bad' cholesterol. What about the good stuff, the kind that's supposed to help prevent plaque build-up?**

A   You're talking about high-density lipoprotein (HDL), which contains the least amount of cholesterol. HDL is considered good because it can remove cholesterol from cells and carry it back to the liver, where it can be excreted from the body via bile acids secreted into the intestines. So high levels of HDL indicate that cholesterol is being removed from the body.

   Components in HDL also help to reduce blood clotting and blood-vessel constriction. That means people with high levels of HDL are less likely to form blood clots in their arteries or to have blood-vessel spasms which can squeeze off blood supply.

   In studies, people with high levels of HDL show a lower risk of developing atherosclerosis. And people with low or even borderline levels of HDL may have increased risk, even when total cholesterol levels are normal. We'll talk more about cholesterol levels in Chapter 3.

Overall, studies find that for each 1 per cent increase in HDL cholesterol, there is about a 3 per cent decrease in your risk of coronary heart disease.

Q   **What's considered a good level of HDL to have?**
A   At least 30 mg/dL if your total cholesterol is very low – 180 mg/dL or less. For most people, levels of 35 mg/dL or higher are best. Some people's HDL levels reach 75 mg/dL or higher. In the average man, HDL cholesterol levels range from 40 to 50 mg/dL; in the average woman, from 50 to 60.

OTHER RISK FACTORS FOR HEART DISEASE

Q   **Aren't there other things besides high cholesterol that are just as bad for your heart? Like smoking, for instance?**
A   Yes. Keep in mind that high cholesterol is only one among many risk factors for heart disease and that it's really only a risk factor, not a disease in itself. For some people, unless cholesterol is very high, it is not even their strongest risk factor for heart disease.

Q   **What are the other risk factors?**
A   Doctors divide them into two categories: those that can't be changed and those you can do something about.

Q   **What are the risk factors you can't change?**
A   Your age, being male rather than female, and having a

family history of premature heart disease — before age 55 in men and age 65 in women.

Q How does your age affect your risk of heart disease?

A The older you are, the greater your risk, no matter what your cholesterol level.

Although risk for heart disease increases continuously with age, heart attacks, angina and other signs of atherosclerosis are relatively rare until age 45 in men and age 55 in women. After that, they increase progressively. For instance, the chance that a 62-year-old man will die of heart disease in the next year is 500 times that of a 22-year-old man. High-cholesterol problems in older people are discussed in Chapter 4.

Q How does gender affect risk of heart disease?

A Men are at higher risk because, until the menopause, a woman is protected from heart disease by the female oestrogen hormones. That's why men in their forties are four times more likely to die of heart disease than are women of the same age. After the menopause, however, a woman's risk increases; but it's still never as high as a man's risk. At age 70, a man is still twice as likely as a woman to die of heart disease. We talk more about women and heart disease in Chapter 4.

Q And what if you have a family history of premature heart disease?

A Your risk of heart disease does increase, but by just how much is uncertain. Some studies show as much as a twelve-fold increase in risk, others only about 25 per cent. A study by researchers at Harvard Medical School found that your risk of heart disease doubles if either your mother or father had a heart attack before age 70, and that your risk increases even more the younger your parent was when he or she had the heart attack. Inherited cholesterol problems are discussed in more detail in Chapter 4.

Q **What are the risk factors you can change?**
A These include cigarette smoking, high blood pressure, lack of exercise, obesity, diabetes, stress and, of course, high cholesterol.

Q **In that order? Are they ranked according to how much of a risk they present?**
A Only roughly. Smoking, high cholesterol, uncontrolled high blood pressure and lack of exercise are considered major risks, but all kinds of variables come into play – how long you've smoked and how much, for instance, or how high your cholesterol or blood pressure is. The same goes for the minor risk factors: obesity, stress and diabetes.

Q **How do these other risk factors stack up against high cholesterol when it comes to a person's risk of developing heart disease?**
A Here again, many variables must be considered. It's possible, however, to make some generalizations. For instance, smokers are $2^1/_2$ times more likely than non-smokers to

have a heart attack. That risk is comparable to what your risk would be if your cholesterol level was 300 mg/dL or so. We'll talk more about smoking in Chapter 7.

Q **And what about high blood pressure? How does it increase your risk of heart disease?**

A As your blood pressure rises from normal (roughly 120/70 mmHg) to between 140/90 and 159/100, your risk of dying of a heart attack or stroke doubles. If it gets to between 160/100 and 179/109 mmHg, your risk trebles.

Q **And diabetes?**

A All else being equal, the risk of heart disease is increased five times in a diabetic woman and two times in a man. There is still no positive decision, however, on the question of whether careful control of blood-sugar levels can decrease these cardiovascular risks. The probability is that it can.

Q **And obesity?**

A It's excess fat, not body weight alone, which seems to increase risk. Excess fat is best measured by something called Body Mass Index (BMI), which is, simply, your weight in kilograms divided by the square of your height in metres.

Here's a quick conversion to help you to determine your BMI: first determine your weight in kilograms. One kilogram is equal to 2.2 pounds, so you must divide your weight in pounds by 2.2 (one stone = 14 pounds, or

6.36 kg). Next you must determine your height in metres. One inch is equal to .0254 metres, so you must multiply your height in inches by .0254. Now take your height as measured in metres and square it – that is, multiply it by itself. Finally, divide your weight in kilograms by this square of your height in metres. The resulting number is your BMI.

In one study, women with a BMI greater than or equal to 29 had almost double the risk of heart disease compared with women with a BMI of less than 21. We talk more about body weight and heart disease in Chapter 7.

Q **How does high cholesterol interact with these other risk factors?**

A The risks are multiplied by any combination of risk factors, including cholesterol. For instance, if you simply smoke cigarettes, you have a 4.6 chance in 100 of having a heart attack within the next eight years. If you smoke *and* have high cholesterol, your chances are 6.4 in 100. And if you *also* have high blood pressure, your chances are about 9.5 in 100.

That's why people with high cholesterol need to look at their other risk factors for heart disease – so they can develop a plan to reduce the overall risk, not just the high cholesterol.

It's true, there's nothing you can do about growing older, being male or having a genetic risk of heart disease. But the more unchangeable risk factors you have, the more likely you are to benefit, perhaps in the near future, by working on the risk factors you *can* change.

In Chapter 2 we look at studies which show just how much of a risk for heart disease high cholesterol has proved to be.

CHAPTER TWO

HIGH CHOLESTEROL
AND HEART DISEASE

STUDIES LINKING HIGH
CHOLESTEROL AND
ATHEROSCLEROSIS

Q **You said earlier that studies show an association between high cholesterol and heart disease. What can you tell me about these studies?**

A Both animal studies and studies of people suggest a strong link between high cholesterol and atherosclerosis, or heart disease.

In 1908 a Russian researcher first noted the connection in rabbits. Later, studies of monkeys demonstrated the direct relationship between cholesterol and saturated fat in the diet, cholesterol levels in the blood and the development of atherosclerosis.

In one such study, for instance, a group of monkeys was fed a typical Western-world diet high in total fat, saturated fat and cholesterol, while another group was fed a prudent diet lower in fat. The animals on the former diet had significantly higher levels of blood cholesterol and much more atherosclerosis in their coronary arteries than those on the prudent diet.

Q   **What about human studies?**

A   Human studies have pretty much confirmed the connection between high blood-cholesterol levels and increased risk of atherosclerosis. They've also confirmed the link between diets high in saturated fat and high cholesterol levels.

For instance, as early as the 1960s medical researchers determined that not all countries had the same amount of atherosclerosis in their populations. Countries with the most heart disease, such as Britain, the US and Norway, had higher average blood-cholesterol levels and consumed more fat than countries with a low rate of heart disease, such as Japan.

Q   **Any more recent studies?**

A   A number of major studies have looked at the link between blood levels of cholesterol and the risk of heart disease in humans.

One of these, the American Multiple Risk Factor Intervention Trial (MRFIT), which ended in 1986, found a strong relationship between blood-cholesterol levels and death from coronary heart disease. For six years the study followed 361,662 men, aged 35 to 57, with no history of heart attack.

This study found that the risk of death from coronary heart disease begins to increase gradually at blood-cholesterol levels of 180 mg/dL, accelerates at about 200 mg/dL, doubles at about 220 mg/dL (in comparison to 180 mg/dL and below) and trebles at about 245 mg/dL. We talk more about cholesterol levels and ranges in Chapter 3.

In this study, the bad effects of high cholesterol were isolated from other major risk factors, such as high blood pressure and cigarette smoking. Doing this helped to establish that high cholesterol, by itself, is a risk factor for atherosclerosis, at least in middle-aged men.

Q   **Any other important studies?**

A   One worth mentioning is the world-famous Framingham Heart Study, which found that, at any age, heart attack rates rise 2 per cent for each 1 per cent increase in blood cholesterol, starting at about 200 mg/dL. People with blood-cholesterol levels of 200 mg/dL or lower had about a 10 per cent risk of coronary artery disease, while people with levels of 240 mg/dL or higher had an 18 per cent risk.

That means 1 out of 10 people with cholesterol lower than 200 mg/dL, and about 2 out of 10 people with cholesterol higher than 240 mg/dL, will develop heart disease.

Q   **Have any studies found no connection between high cholesterol levels and heart disease?**

A   There are some which show only a weak link. Just how strong a connection is found depends on lots of factors: the people being studied, the length of the study and the means used to determine heart disease. Links between cholesterol and heart disease are weaker in women, especially pre-menopausal women, and in both men and women over the age of 70. Also, researchers now know that total cholesterol is not as good a predictor of heart disease as are some other cholesterol measurements, such as HDL-to-LDL ratio, which we talk about more in Chapter 3.

Q Wasn't there a recent study which showed that people over a certain age needn't worry if their cholesterol is high?

A Yes. One study found that high cholesterol may not be as good a predictor of heart disease in people aged 70 or older as it is in younger people. We talk more about what older people need to know about high cholesterol in Chapter 4.

PROOF THAT LOWER CHOLESTEROL MEANS LESS HEART DISEASE

Q OK, you've presented evidence to show that high blood levels of cholesterol are associated with an increased risk of heart disease. But is there proof that lowering cholesterol levels reduces a person's risk?

A Yes. Most of the 20 or more studies which have looked at this question have shown a significant reduction in the incidence of coronary heart disease after blood-cholesterol levels were lowered, either through diet alone or with diet and drugs.

Many of the studies using cholesterol-lowering drugs failed to show a reduction in total deaths, however, and some showed an increase. This is a disturbing finding which we discuss in more detail below and in Chapter 4.

Q **What can you tell me about the studies which show that lowering cholesterol reduces a person's risk of heart disease?**

A One of the earliest, the Lipid Research Clinics Coronary Primary Prevention Trial, included 3,806 healthy middle-aged men with high levels of total blood cholesterol and LDL cholesterol; they were followed for seven years during the 1970s.

All the men followed a reduced-fat diet and also took either a cholesterol-lowering drug called **cholestyramine** or a placebo (inactive drug) which looked just like it. The men taking the cholestyramine decreased their total cholesterol by 11.8 per cent and their LDL cholesterol by 18.9 per cent. They also had a slight increase in HDL cholesterol. The men taking the placebo had reductions of 5 per cent in total cholesterol and 8.6 per cent in LDL.

Deaths from heart attacks were almost 20 per cent less in the men taking cholestyramine compared with the men taking the placebo. At cholesterol levels above 200 mg/dL, for each 1 per cent reduction of blood cholesterol and LDL cholesterol there was a 2 per cent reduction in coronary heart disease. There was also a similar reduction in **angina pectoris** and in the need for coronary artery bypass surgery. And **electrocardiography** tests, which measure and record electrical activity in the heart, detected fewer signs of coronary artery blockages in the people whose cholesterol was lowered.

Q **Do other studies show similar results?**

A Yes, they tend to. Another notable study, with results published in 1987, was the Helsinki Heart Study. This five-year trial included more than 4,000 healthy, middle-aged Finnish men. The men did not have evidence of heart disease, but they did have high blood levels of LDL cholesterol and **very low-density lipoprotein (VLDL)** cholesterol. They received either the cholesterol-lowering drug **gemfibrozil** (Lopid) or a placebo.

In the group taking the drug there was a significant reduction in total cholesterol (10 per cent) and LDL cholesterol (11 per cent), and an 11 per cent increase in HDL. Compared with a control group taking a placebo, there were 34 per cent fewer new cases of angina or heart attacks in the men taking gemfibrozil.

CHOLESTEROL-LOWERING IN PEOPLE WITH HEART DISEASE

Q **What about people who already have signs of athero-sclerosis? Do studies show that lowering cholesterol helps them to avoid a heart attack?**

A Most do. For instance, the Coronary Drug Project, done in the early and mid-1970s, used two medications: **nicotinic acid** (a form of **niacin**, a vitamin) and **clofibrate** (Atromid-S). (Two other drugs, dextrothyroxine and oestrogen, were dropped from this study because of serious side-effects.)

This study involved men who already had coronary heart disease. Half were treated with either of these cholesterol-lowering drugs; half were treated with a placebo. The purpose was to see if heart disease was less likely to recur in the men treated with the drugs.

In comparison to the placebo group, the incidence of coronary heart disease was almost 20 per cent less in men taking nicotinic acid; it was 9.5 per cent less in the men taking clofibrate. Even in these men, for each 1 per cent decrease in blood cholesterol there was about a 2 per cent decrease in recurrence of coronary heart disease – the same reduction in risk of heart disease as other studies found for people with no apparent signs of heart disease.

Q Any other studies I should know about?

A Yes. The Stockholm Ischaemic Heart Disease Secondary Prevention Study, which ended in 1988, involved heart attack survivors who took a combination of either clofibrate and nicotinic acid, or clofibrate and a placebo, for five years. At the end of that time the people taking the two drugs had a 13 per cent drop in cholesterol and a 36 per cent reduction in deaths from coronary artery disease.

Q Anything newer than that?

A The latest study, the Scandinavian Simvastatin Survival Study ('4-S' for short), was conducted at 94 medical centres in Denmark, Finland, Iceland, Norway and Sweden. It found that people previously diagnosed with atherosclerosis who took the cholesterol-lowering drug **simvastatin** (Zocor) were only about half as likely to die of a heart attack as people taking a placebo. In addition, chances of having a non-fatal heart attack or of requiring surgery to open or bypass blocked arteries were cut by about one-third in people taking simvastatin. Incidentally, both groups also ate a reduced-fat diet.

This study, completed in 1994, involved 4,444 men and women aged 35 to 70, with cholesterol levels of 212 to 309 mg/dL. They were followed up for an average of about 5 1/2 years.

Many doctors consider this an important study because it is the first cholesterol-lowering study to show a reduction in overall death rates, not just deaths from heart attacks. People taking the drug were about one-third less likely to die prematurely of a cause other than heart disease.

LOWER CHOLESTEROL MIGHT NOT MEAN LONGER LIFE

Q   **Are you saying that the other studies before this didn't find that lowering cholesterol helped people live longer?**

A   Yes, that's exactly what we're saying. Even though lowering cholesterol helped to reduce deaths from heart disease and related problems, a number of studies have found that men with very low cholesterol – usually

160 mg/dL or below – were more likely than men with normal cholesterol levels to die of causes other than heart disease.

Q **What were these men dying of?**
A A variety of causes, including accidents, suicides and gall-bladder and liver problems.

Q **Well, we've all got to die of something, right?**
A Yes, but that doesn't explain this finding. These were premature deaths, and it's hard to explain them. The link between low cholesterol and death has been investigated.

Q **Do researchers think that low cholesterol caused these deaths?**
A No one knows for sure. One class of cholesterol-lowering drugs, **fibric acid derivatives** – clofibrate and gemfibrozil – may have contributed to the deaths. (We talk more about these drugs in Chapter 6.) But researchers are also looking into the possibility that low cholesterol levels may change hormone levels in a way that contributes to health problems, including depression and compulsive behaviour. That's something we look at in more detail in Chapter 4.

One other thing you should realize: statistical findings of studies are sometimes cited in a way that makes the potential benefit of cholesterol-lowering appear greater than it really is in some cases, especially for people who haven't got heart disease.

RELATIVE, ABSOLUTE AND ATTRIBUTABLE RISK

Q What do you mean?

A Take the Helsinki Heart Study just mentioned, for instance, although you could do the same thing with any study. In that study, the researchers concluded that five years of treatment with a cholesterol-lowering drug resulted in a 34 per cent reduction in the risk of non-fatal heart attacks and death caused by coronary artery disease.

**Q Well, that seems straightforward enough. What's the
A problem?**

Bear with us a moment and look at the actual figures. In the control group of 2,030 people, there were 84 coronary heart disease events (a rate of 4.1 per cent); in the treatment group of 2,050 people, there were 56 coronary heart disease events (a rate of 2.7 per cent).

Q So what's the problem?

A Well, the reduction in actual risk, or absolute risk, as it's called in statistics, is only 1.4 per cent (4.1 minus 2.7). That means that if 100 people took a cholesterol-lowering drug for five years, only 1.4 coronary events, such as heart attacks, would be prevented. It means that 98.6 people would be taking a cholesterol-lowering drug, and exposing themselves to the possible risks associated with taking that drug, without seeing any benefit.

Q **But what about the 34 per cent reduction?**

A That figure is the **relative risk** reduction, a comparison of the risks between two different groups. In this case, researchers take the difference in risk between the control group and treatment group (1.4 per cent) and divide it by the risk in the control group (4.1 per cent.) While that figure may be relevant to public health officials trying to decide how many fewer people will develop a particular disease as a result of some sort of intervention, it's not especially helpful to individuals who are trying to decide the best way to allocate their limited time, money and energy in terms of good health.

Q **I think I see what you mean, but could you say it again?**

A People like to know their odds, or chances of something happening, before they make big decisions or take risks. They also like to know how these odds can be changed.

For instance, let's say you are told your risk of having a heart attack in the next five years is 5 in 10. (That's the total absolute risk.) You're also told that if you stop smoking, your odds will drop to 3 in 10; that if you also get your cholesterol down to 200 mg/dL, your odds will be 2 in 10; and if you can, in addition to all the above things, get your blood pressure down to normal, your odds will be 1 in 10. You can see exactly how each one of these changes affects your actual, or absolute risk.

Q **Do researchers have any other special names for types of risk?**

A The amount of risk that can be specifically blamed on a

risk factor, such as smoking, researchers call the **attribut-able risk**. In the previous example, the attributable risk reduction of smoking is 2: the absolute risk (5), less the risk if you stop smoking (3). The attributable risk reduction of both cholesterol-lowering and blood pressure control is 1 each.

Q   **Is knowing the attributable risk important?**

A   Yes. It can help you to work out which health risk factors are increasing your total risk most and, therefore, which are most important for you to change. It lets you know which interventions are going to give you the most benefit – reduction in risk – for your efforts.

   By measuring relative and absolute risk in large groups of people, studies such as the Helsinki one ultimately help doctors to weigh each individual's attributable and absolute risks.

Q   **How am I supposed to determine my absolute risk for something?**

A   Ask your GP. When your GP prescribes a treatment, ask him or her to tell you exactly how much difference it can really make for you. If it's a cholesterol-lowering drug that's being prescribed, ask questions – what are your chances of having a heart attack if you don't take the drug? What are your chances if you do decide to take the drug? Find out about the *real* benefits for you.

CHAPTER THREE

CHOLESTEROL TESTING

GUIDELINES FOR CHOLESTEROL TESTING

Q Who should have their cholesterol measured?

A   The answer will depend on whom you ask. In the US, the general recommendation – based on the views of the American Medical Association and the American College of Cardiology – is that anyone aged 20 or older should have his or her total cholesterol and HDL cholesterol measured at least once every five years. Many British doctors are less enthusiastic about routine testing.

Q How about young children? Do they need to have their cholesterol checked?

A   Paediatricians normally don't check a child's cholesterol until at least age two. After that age, testing is routinely done only for children with a family history of premature heart disease (heart attack before age 55) or other apparent risk factors, such as severe obesity. One reason you might have a child's cholesterol checked as early as this is to detect rare but serious inherited cholesterol disorders which can lead to problems, including heart disease, early in life. See Chapter 4 for more on children and inherited cholesterol disorders.

Q   **And teenagers – when should they be tested?**
A   A teenager's cholesterol levels might be checked any time if he or she has never been checked previously, especially if there is a family history of premature heart disease or other risk factors, such as smoking, obesity or high blood pressure.

Q   **If I already know I have high cholesterol, should I have it checked more often?**
A   Guidelines vary as to when you should have your cholesterol re-checked. It depends on your levels of different lipoproteins, the number of risk factors you have for heart disease and how aggressively you're trying to lower your cholesterol. Your best bet is to ask your GP.

Q   **What exactly does a cholesterol test measure?**
A   If the test involves taking a few drops of blood from your fingertip, it can measure total cholesterol and sometimes HDL cholesterol. But if tubes of blood are taken from a vein in your arm (called venous blood), more things can be measured in the blood – total cholesterol, HDL and triglycerides. (LDL cholesterol is measured indirectly, by subtracting other components from your total cholesterol.)

Q   **If they're measuring all those things, is it still called a cholesterol test?**

A   Your GP might call it that, but technically this test is called a **complete lipid profile**.

Q   **Is that the kind of blood test I'd have to fast for?**

A   Yes. It's possible to get fairly accurate measurements of total cholesterol and HDL cholesterol even if you've eaten recently, since these lipids don't change much with a meal. But triglycerides and LDL cholesterol are influenced by what you've just eaten. Their levels start to rise within an hour or two of a meal, and stay elevated for 12 hours or so.

To eliminate this as an influence on your cholesterol reading, you'll be told to fast (go without eating) for about 12 hours. Usually you are told not to eat anything after 6 p.m. the night before the test. Then the blood is drawn first thing next morning.

Q   **What happens if I do eat something?**

A   Even having as little as a cup of coffee with milk can affect the results, so you should obey the 'nil by mouth' rule. If you forget and have something to eat, arrange to have the test on another day.

PROBLEMS WITH ACCURACY

Q   I've heard that those finger-prick tests offered at shops and health exhibitions or fairs aren't very accurate. Are they?

A   No one knows. There is no way to check their accuracy or to determine that the equipment being used is properly calibrated. You can rely on proper hospital and most other medical laboratories, but 'freelance' testing is less certain.

Q   Does that mean I shouldn't bother to have this sort of test done?

A   That's up to you, but you shouldn't consider the results reliable. Whether the results are high, low or in between, you shouldn't rely on them as the only measurement of your cholesterol.

Q   What about at-home cholesterol testing kits? Are they any more accurate than shop testing?

A   Again, there is doubt. This is not really a matter for DIY. Most doctors would agree that the interpretation and validity of the at-home tests are open to serious question, and that they should not be relied upon as your only source of information about your cholesterol. Commercial blood-cholesterol analysers currently range in price from £2,995 to £13,730, so in all probability a home kit costing less than £200 will not be such a bargain.

Q   **Why would someone use one of these tests?**
A   Good question. Unlike the home tests used by diabetic
    people for monitoring blood sugar, cholesterol tests
    usually do not need to be done quickly or often.
        People might use one to screen themselves for high
    cholesterol, just as might be done at a health fair. Or if
    they're trying to reduce their cholesterol with diet,
    weight loss or drugs, they might use it between visits to
    the surgery to satisfy their own curiosity as to how well
    they're doing.

Q   **These tests use so little blood. How do they work?**
A   The blood reacts with chemical-impregnated filter paper.
    A chemical in the paper converts cholesterol to hydro-
    gen peroxide. The more cholesterol, the more hydrogen
    peroxide produced. The filter paper then soaks up the
    hydrogen peroxide, and your cholesterol 'reading'
    depends on how far along the paper the hydrogen
    peroxide has been drawn. A scale alongside the paper
    gives your reading. You can put too much blood into
    one of these tests and still get an accurate reading, since
    excess blood is squeezed off. But too little blood will give
    you a falsely low reading.

Q   **Is a doctor's cholesterol testing any better than health-
    fair or at-home tests?**
A   It's possible that you can get a more accurate reading at
    a GP's consulting room than at a health fair. But again,
    there is no way to know that for sure. Of course, if the

doctor takes blood from a vein and sends it to a hospital laboratory, you can absolutely rely on the result.

Q **So hospital laboratories are licenced and regulated?**
A Certainly. They are under strict regulations. They require proficiency testing to prove that the equipment works properly and that the staff know how to use it. However, no one actually monitors the accuracy of testing in GPs' consulting rooms. That would be impracticable, given the variety of instruments and techniques used by doctors to measure cholesterol. Many doctors don't do it at all, relying instead on official laboratories.

The American experience on this matter is interesting. A 1995 report from the Federal General Accounting Office found that the tabletop analysers used to measure cholesterol in about 19 per cent of doctors' offices and at most health-fair cholesterol screenings have an error rate of 17 to 50 per cent. Some of the doctors' offices had their own small clinical laboratories, and instead of using tabletop analysers used smaller versions of the same sort of analysers used at large professional laboratories.

Q **What if my doctor sends my blood to a hospital laboratory for analysis? How accurate will that be?**
A Perfectly adequate. You can count on an accuracy of better than plus or minus 8.9 per cent.

Q **What other kinds of things can interfere with a cholesterol test's accuracy?**
A All sorts of things, especially you, can have an impact on

your cholesterol test. The main source of variation in the result and in misinterpretation of a cholesterol test is not the laboratory, it is you.

Q **What causes this variation in cholesterol levels in people?**

A Your body can. A reading may change depending on whether blood is drawn from a capillary or a vein, whether you are standing or seated, the composition of recent meals, whether you've been ill recently, if you're pregnant or taking drugs, whether you are losing or gaining weight, even the time of year. (Cholesterol tends to be slightly lower during the summer months.)

THE BEST WAY TO TEST

Q **So what does all this mean? Are you suggesting that I shouldn't even bother to have my cholesterol tested?**

A No, but have it done correctly. Here are some suggestions:

- Make sure that your weight, diet and all the medication you are taking have been unchanged for at least four months.
- Have the test performed on a sample of blood drawn from a vein, usually in your arm, not capillary blood from a finger-prick.
- Limit your physical activity to quiet walking before the test, and sit quietly for 10 to 15 minutes before the sample is drawn.

- Don't allow a tourniquet to remain on your arm for more than 30 to 60 seconds before blood is drawn.
- Have your sample sent to a hospital laboratory for analysis.

Q   So if I do all these things, am I assured of accurate results?

A   You're as close as you're going to get.

Q   So is that all I need to do?

A   Possibly. If you follow the above advice and your total cholesterol reading is lower than 180 mg/dL, you can safely assume that, so far as blood cholesterol is concerned, you are not at increased risk of heart disease and need no further testing at the time. Your HDL should also be higher than 35 mg/dL.

Q   What if my cholesterol reading is higher than that?

A   The trouble is that if your total cholesterol is above 180 mg/dL, the variation is great enough that you don't really know what risk group you are in. Your average, day-to-day value could be higher than 200 mg/dL. So you'll want to wait three or four weeks (to help minimize the impact of seasonal variations in cholesterol), then have a repeat test, done at the same laboratory and in the same manner.

Q   What's that supposed to do?

A   You can compare the two results to see how close they are. If the first two readings are within 15 per cent of each other, you can average the two and use that figure as your guide. In other words, if one reading is 210 mg/dL and another is 240 mg/dL, add them together, divide by two, and come up with 225 mg/dL as your nominal cholesterol level.

Q   **What if the two readings are far apart?**

A   If the second result differs by more than 15 per cent from the first, review your health status and pre-test preparation period. Were there any changes? If not, get a third reading, again waiting three to four weeks.

Q   **Now, what do I do with the three numbers?**

A   Throw out the one that's furthest from the other two and average the two that are within 15 per cent of each other. If no two are within 15 per cent of each other, either your health status, the pre-test preparation or the blood-drawing and sample-handling processes are not uniform. This is unusual, so try to decide what variations could be affecting your results before beginning again.

Q   **If my initial cholesterol reading is high, should I also go through this additional testing?**

A   If your total cholesterol is 240 mg/dL or higher, you should get a second reading, but don't wait to get a second test to begin to do something about it. You really shouldn't need the stimulus of a high cholesterol reading to start losing weight, to give up smoking and start exercising. However, any decision to start taking cholesterol-lowering drugs should be based on more than one measurement.

Q   **What about checking my HDL and LDL levels? Is that important?**
A   Yes. Most doctors believe it's important for anyone with a total cholesterol reading of 200 mg/dL or higher (some doctors even say as low as 180 mg/dL) to have their HDL, LDL and triglyceride levels measured.

Q   **Why are these other measurements so important?**
A   They take into account the breakdown of cholesterol in your blood, not just the total amount. In other words, they seem to give a more accurate assessment of your real risk of developing heart disease than does total cholesterol alone, experts say.

Q   **How so?**
A   The fact is that most of the people who have heart attacks haven't got exceptionally high cholesterol readings. They have cholesterol levels between 200 and 250 mg/dL, just like most people. So what is needed is to identify the people at highest risk of heart attacks.

Q   **How is that done?**
A   All of a person's risk factors need to be considered – whether he or she is overweight, diabetic, smokes or has a strong family history of heart disease, for instance.

In addition to this, doctors will want to know a person's levels of HDL and LDL cholesterol and, usually, triglycerides, because each of these blood components is considered to carry its own risks for heart disease.

HDL AND LDL LEVELS AND RATIOS

Q   **What's considered a good level of HDL cholesterol?**

A   Anything below 35 mg/dL has been found to increase a person's risk of heart disease, although some people with very low total cholesterol (160 mg/dL or lower) have an HDL level below 35 mg/dL with no apparent increased risk. Levels of 35 to 50 or so are considered normal, but some people's HDL can reach 75 mg/dL or higher. In several large studies, a 1 mg/dL increase in HDL cholesterol was associated with a 2 to 3 per cent decrease in risk of coronary heart disease.

Q   **And what levels of LDL cholesterol are good?**

A   Amounts less than 130 mg/dL are considered desirable, and amounts less than 100 mg/dL are associated with a reversal of coronary heart disease. Borderline high levels are 130 to 149 mg/dL; anything over 150 mg/dL is high.

Q   **How do doctors juggle all these figures?**

A   One thing they sometimes do is come up with ratios of one blood lipid to another. Researchers, especially, are looking at ratios because they appear to be better predictors of heart disease than is total cholesterol alone.

Q   **What kind of ratios do they use?**

A   Total-cholesterol-to-HDL is one ratio that seems to help pinpoint risks. In studies, a total-cholesterol-to-HDL ratio of less than 6:1 seems to protect against heart disease, while a ratio greater than 6:1 predisposes to heart disease.

Some doctors also determine LDL-to-HDL ratios. In studies, an LDL-to-HDL ratio of less than 4:1 is protective, whereas a ratio higher than 4:1 is predisposing to heart disease.

Q   **My doctor never mentioned ratios to me. Can I work this out on my own?**

A   Yes, if you know your total cholesterol, HDL and LDL. Your total-cholesterol-to-HDL ratio is simply total cholesterol divided by HDL. The same goes for LDL-to-HDL. Simply divide the first figure by the second.

Q   **Does any ratio stand out as being a particularly good predictor of coronary artery disease?**

A   So far, total-cholesterol-to-HDL seems to be the best predictor. But experts disagree on the value of ratios, and some say ratios can be misleading and that you should always look at the figures themselves, too.

TRIGLYCERIDE LEVELS

Q   **What about triglycerides? When should they be measured?**

A   Doctors say you should have your triglycerides measured if you find you have total cholesterol higher than 200 mg/dL, if you have two or more coronary heart disease risk factors, diabetes, high blood pressure, kidney disease or a condition called **pancreatitis** (inflammation of the pancreas).

Q **What are considered good levels of triglycerides?**

A Normal levels are less than 200 mg/dL; borderline high, 200 to 400 mg/dL; high, 400 to 1,000 mg/dL and very high, 1,000 mg/dL or above.

Q **That's enough about figures. What does all this mean to me, the patient?**

A The point is this: your doctor is going to use the results of your cholesterol tests to help make decisions regarding your medical treatment. You want to make sure he or she is working with accurate figures and that he or she knows how to interpret these numbers. So ask for a copy of your cholesterol test. Know your total cholesterol, your HDL, LDL and triglyceride levels. Check Table A on page 41 to see what risk categories you fall into. And check Table B on page 42 to see what other risk factors for coronary heart disease you have.

Ask your doctor to explain his or her treatment decisions, and what they are based on.

And remember, high cholesterol by itself is not a 'disease'. It's simply one among many risk factors for heart disease.

TABLE A

Total cholesterol

Desirable	Less than 200 mg/dL
Borderline high	200–239 mg/dL
High	240 mg/dL or higher

HDL cholesterol

Desirable	50–75 mg/dL or higher
Borderline low	35—49 mg/dL
Low	Less than 35 mg/dL

LDL cholesterol

Desirable	Less than 130 mg/dL
Borderline high	130–149 mg/dL
High	150 mg/dL or higher

Triglycerides

Safe	200 mg/dL or less
Borderline high	200–400 mg/dL
High	400–1,000 mg/dL
Very high	1,000 mg/dL or above

TABLE B

Additional Risk Factors for Coronary Heart Disease
High cholesterol is only one risk factor for coronary
artery disease. These additional risk factors are just as
important:

- Age 45 or older in men
- Age 55 or older in women
- Cigarette smoking
- Diabetes mellitus (noninsulin-dependent, or
  adult-onset)
- HDL less than 35 mg/dL
- History of **cerebrovascular disease** (stroke) or
  occlusive peripheral vascular disease (intermit-
  tent claudication)
- High blood pressure
- LDL 130 mg/dL or higher
- Heart attack or sudden death before age 55 in a
  parent or sibling
- Severe obesity (30 per cent or more over ideal
  weight)
- Total cholesterol 200 mg/dL or more

CHAPTER FOUR

SPECIAL INTEREST GROUPS

WOMEN AND CHOLESTEROL

Q I just had my cholesterol checked and it was 250 mg/dL. The doctor says this is OK because I am a woman. What does she mean?

A Your doctor may be referring to results from the ongoing, two-decade long Framingham Heart Study, one of the few cholesterol-monitoring studies to include women. Researchers found that what's considered a high total cholesterol level for men – and therefore an important risk indicator for heart disease – does not correlate to women. In general, women do not begin to have heart disease-related problems, such as heart attacks, until their cholesterol levels reach 265 mg/dL. That's 25 mg/dL above the danger zone for men, which begins at 240 mg/dL.

Q Does this mean women can tolerate higher levels of cholesterol and can relax about buttering toast?

A Sorry, there's no indication that women are free to binge

on butter or other artery-clogging foods without suffer-
ing cholesterol consequences. What seems clear is that
women normally have higher overall cholesterol levels
than men because of the positive effects of the female
hormone oestrogen, not because they can tolerate more
plaque-building cholesterol in their arteries.

Q Why? What has oestrogen got that's so helpful?
A Oestrogen boosts the production of HDL, the cholesterol that escorts fat from the bloodstream and slows
plaque build-up in the artery walls, which is caused by
LDL. Thanks to oestrogen, women, on average, have an
HDL level of 55 mg/dL compared with an average of
45 mg/dL for men. In short, their oestrogen edge gives
women built-in heart-disease protection – at least until
the menopause.

Q Then what happens?
A Once a woman reaches the menopause and oestrogen
levels naturally decline, HDL cholesterol production
drops. And there goes the natural protection against
plaque build-up. The Framingham people found that if
HDL levels dip – even a little – a woman's heart-disease
risk rises greatly. And in the Lipid Research Clinic's
Follow-up Study, women who had as little as a 10 mg/dL
drop in HDL doubled their risk of heart disease. One
proven method women can use to compensate for this
drop is to take oestrogen-replacement hormones, a
course known as hormone replacement therapy (HRT).

Q You mean I could have low total cholesterol but still be at risk of heart disease because my HDL level is also low?

A Absolutely. To determine if that 250 mg/dL cholesterol reading of yours is really safe, you need to know your HDL level, which provides a more precise indicator of heart-disease risk than total cholesterol alone. But you can't ignore your LDL either. While these 'bad' lipids do not seem to be as important predictors of heart disease in women as they are in men, LDLs are still the bodies that lay down the plaque on arteries, and their effect can't be completely neutralized by HDLs.

Q So how high should my HDLs be? How low should my LDLs be?

A As a general rule of thumb, women should have HDLs higher than 55 mg/dL and LDLs of lower than 130 mg/dL. With that said, however, the Framingham Study indicates that it's more precise to know the ratio of total cholesterol to HDLs in your blood. As we explained in Chapter 3, ideally the ratio of total cholesterol to HDL levels should not exceed 6:1. If you are above that your risk of heart disease soars. Furthermore, your LDL-to-HDL ratio should not exceed 4:1. These same safe ratios, by the way, also apply to men.

Q I'm getting bogged down in figures. Can you review this ratio business again?

A If your total cholesterol reading is 250, for example, then your HDL should be 50 or more to stay within the recommended 6:1 safe zone. If your LDL is 140, then your HDL should be 35 or higher, so as not to exceed the 4:1 safe zone.

Q   **OK, so I should know my HDLs and LDLs and not worry about the total cholesterol?**

A   Not exactly. The Framingham Study showed that women under the age of 50 who had the highest total-cholesterol levels were most likely to develop heart disease.

Until there's more conclusive data on women and heart disease, most experts advise you to keep your total cholesterol at 200 mg/dL or less, no matter what your sex. This involves reducing the amount of high-fat foods in your diet, exercising, and controlling other risk factors such as weight gain and smoking. Smoking, by the way, reduces oestrogen levels, lowers HDLs and raises LDLs, prompts the onset of early menopause, and shifts body-fat distribution to your waistline. This fat shift creates an 'apple' shape, which is associated with higher LDLs. Smoking is too dangerous altogether.

Q   **My doctor told me that triglyceride levels really deter-mine a woman's heart-disease risk. Is that true?**

A   Triglycerides are blood fats that come from the diet or are made in the liver. And it's true, their link with heart disease is stronger in women than it is in men. While the role of triglycerides is still uncertain, their significance to women's heart-disease risk appears to be a case of 'guilt by association' with HDLs. Both lipids are affected by oestrogen. Studies have shown that after the menopause, when oestrogen wanes, HDL levels drop sharply while triglycerides rise, which is bad news. Studies also show that when women take synthetic oestrogen (HRT), HDL levels rise, but so do triglycerides. Some researchers believe that synthetic oestrogen may alter HDL, making it less able to remove cholesterol. (By the way, HRT which also includes **progesterone** appears to raise triglycerides less significantly.)

While studies show a connection between HDLs and triglycerides, the connection to developing heart disease remains unclear. Some experts say that high triglycerides are a marker, or an indicator, of an underlying problem in processing blood fats, possibly due to oestrogen preparations or other medications, or diabetes, which puts a person at increased risk of coronary heart disease.

Indeed, the Framingham Study shows that high triglyceride levels (above 190 mg/dL) are premier predictors of heart disease in women, particularly post-menopausal women, but not in men. In younger women, the oestrogen hormone may override any potential harm or produce a more benign form of triglycerides. In any case, to get a true picture of your cholesterol as well as your risk, get the complete lipid figures – including triglyceride levels.

Q   **At what age should women be tested for cholesterol?**
A   Some doctors suggest that, in general, women with a family history of heart disease should have a lipid profile test done before the age of 18 and be closely monitored

thereafter. Women without a family history of heart disease should have a complete cholesterol workup at the age of 30 and certainly before the menopause, when lipids change.

Q **Before prescribing the Pill, my doctor wants my cholesterol checked. Why is that?**

A The contraceptive pill has not always been shown to be lipid-friendly. Studies done on earlier, more potent versions of the Pill, which contained high oestrogen doses, showed that Pill-users had a three-fold increase in death from heart disease compared with women not taking the Pill. Studies have also shown that oral contraceptives which contain progesterone can cause blood clots and may also change fat and carbohydrate metabolism. The Pill is a good news/bad news story. The high-dose oestrogen component of earlier versions boosted triglycerides and, more significantly, the good HDLs – but unfortunately, not enough to compensate for the raised LDLs, which got bumped up thanks to the high-dose progesterone component.

Q **What about newer versions of the Pill?**

A The newer, low-dose contraceptive pills, which contain less potent oestrogen and progesterone, appear to increase LDLs only mildly, while increasing HDLs. But you still need a complete cholesterol workup before going on any oral contraceptive. An annual checkup is also necessary. Some doctors rule out the Pill if cholesterol levels exceed 220 mg/dL or triglycerides exceed

190 mg/dL. Other doctors believe that elevated cholesterol or triglyceride levels should not necessarily rule out
Pill use, since the oestrogen component would cancel
out harmful LDLs and triglycerides. However, oral
contraceptives are taboo if you are extremely overweight, smoke or have very high blood pressure.

Q **Let's say I'm menopausal and, since heart disease runs in
my family, my doctor recommends hormone replacement therapy. Is that because it lowers cholesterol?**

A Replacement oestrogen affects cholesterol in two ways:
it increases HDL and decreases LDL, both by 10 to 15
per cent, according to some studies. Post-menopausal
HRT has been shown to cut women's risk of heart
disease in half. But it's not for everyone and it's not the
only weapon in the anti-cholesterol war. Talk to your GP
about diet, exercise and weight control. Read books by
qualified doctors that discuss the HRT question, review
all your risk factors and get a second opinion.

Q **I've heard that the newer versions of HRT reduce
uterine cancer but may cancel out heart protection
and also increase the risk of breast cancer. True or
false?**

A Recent research results may cast HRT in a new, more
favourable light. These show that oestrogen used alone
or in combination with a progestin (synthetic progesterone, added to counteract harmful uterine-tissue build-
up) does not, in fact, block oestrogen's positive effects
on lipids. This HRT combination also improves HDL

levels, although the increase is only slight. If oestrogen alone is used, there is a 5 mg/dL rise in HDLs; if progestin is added, HDLs rise by less than half that amount.

Experts predict that updated HRT formulas with a micronized, gentler form of progestin (similar to the type used in the Pill) will soon be available. These formulas will have even less of a negative impact on the oestrogen's positive effects. In the mean time, experts point out HRT's other heart-healthy benefits: it lowers high blood pressure and protects the arteries. Although the risk of breast cancer does increase – and has had the lion's share of publicity regarding HRT – breast cancer causes far fewer deaths than heart disease, and clearly the advantage of saving thousands of women from early death from heart disease convincingly outweighs the possible risk of breast cancer. According to some doctors, the only post-menopausal women who should be excluded from HRT use are those with a blood clot or liver disease.

Q **Which form of HRT protects better: the patch or the Pill?**

A The Pill – oral contraceptive – lowers cholesterol best, because, as it is taken by mouth, the hormone, like all food, must pass through the liver to be metabolized, so it has a direct effect on liver function. (The liver, you'll recall, makes cholesterol for the rest of the body.)

A skin patch, on the other hand, provides oestrogen directly through the skin and, from there, into the blood-stream. Although some oestrogen does reach the liver, its effects are much reduced. Still, women who use the patch do gain some protection from heart disease. Indeed, the patch may be the preferred method of HRT if you have very high triglyceride levels, since oral oestrogen may raise triglycerides.

CHILDREN AND CHOLESTEROL

Q Our family doctor says it's never too early to start a heart-healthy diet. Just how early does heart disease begin anyway? Are my children at risk?

A Some experts say it's over the top to start children on a low-fat diet unless they're overweight or have extremely high cholesterol. But there is some evidence that, as early as the age of three, arteries may begin developing fatty streaks made up of fat and connective tissue. Apparently, too, the more extensive the streaks in childhood the more likely they are to advance to atherosclerosis.

A few years ago, researchers looked at cholesterol levels of children over a period of 15 years. Autopsies of the children in the study who died accidentally during this time revealed that those who had higher levels of overall cholesterol in earlier years had more extensive fatty streaks in the largest artery in their bodies (the aorta). While there is no definite proof, this and other evidence leads some experts to believe that children with high cholesterol levels are more likely than the general population to have high cholesterol as adults.

Q   **What do fatty streaks have to do with what my child eats?**

A   As explained more fully in Chapter 5, fatty streaks are caused by high blood levels of cholesterol, which usually are a result of eating foods high in saturated fats. Preference for this sort of junk food – burgers, chips and the like – is determined early in life. Unfortunately, the earlier your child starts eating high-fat foods and the more he eats, the more likely it is that he will develop the high-cholesterol levels that put him at risk of heart disease. A high-fat diet is a particularly important risk factor if premature heart disease runs in the family – before age 55 in men and before age 65 in women.

Q   **So how do I know if my child's cholesterol is high?**

A   Most doctors don't routinely screen children for high cholesterol unless one or both parents have high cholesterol. So if you or your partner have a total cholesterol level above 200–240 mg/dL and further tests reveal HDLs lower than 35 mg/dL, LDLs higher than 130 mg/dL or triglycerides above 250 mg/dL, it's time to ask for an initial measurement of total cholesterol for your child. High cholesterol can be passed on from parent to child, and the earlier you identify it and take measures to control it, the less likely it is to progress.

Q   **But my child is not even of school age. Isn't that a bit young for screening tests? What do the tests involve?**

A   She's not too young if there's a family history and if you or your partner's blood levels indicate that she could be at high risk. In this instance, any time after the age of two is acceptable to have her tested for cholesterol. Some experts contend that those children whose parents have high cholesterol should certainly be tested before the age of 10. Some doctors also recommend cholesterol testing for children who are excessively overweight or for teenagers who smoke or use oral contraceptives.

Q   **Does the doctor have to draw blood from a vein?**

A   Perhaps not. Your doctor may first give your child a simple finger-prick blood test. Ideally, the level should be under 170 mg/dL for children aged 2 to 19. Even if it's below this level and you're enthusiastic about it, you will rightly want to limit the burgers, promote exercise and discourage smoking. In five years, your child should be re-checked for cholesterol levels.

Q   **And if my child's cholesterol is high?**

A   There's a one in four chance your child's cholesterol will be higher than 170 mg/dL. A high cholesterol reading means that your child needs a further, more detailed test – the complete lipid profile discussed in Chapter 3. That test involves drawing blood from a vein following a 12-hour fast. A complete lipoprotein analysis is also recommended if either parent or grandparent has documented premature heart disease, such as a heart attack before the age of 55.

Q   It's not so easy keeping children from eating for 12
    hours, let alone getting them to sit still for a needle.
    How important are these tests?

A   Very. It's the only way to assess a child's real risk accu-
    rately. A complete lipid profile can tell you if your child's
    high cholesterol is due to raised HDLs (which is good
    and affects about 15 to 20 per cent of children with high
    overall cholesterol) or if it's due to raised LDLs, the
    artery-clogging lipids. This is not so good, and occurs in 1
    in 20 children. The test can also reveal if your child's
    triglyceride levels exceed the recommended level of 100
    mg/dL for children under the age of 10, or 130 for chil-
    dren over that age.

Q   I take it high triglycerides is a bad sign in children?

A   Yes, as it is in adults. High triglycerides are a tip-off that
    children may have an inherited condition associated with
    premature heart disease, which occurs in 5 per cent of
    children. Basically their bodies are unable to metabolize
    fat.

Q   If early high cholesterol levels might indicate prema-
    ture heart disease, why don't they routinely test for it
    in school?

A   Experts believe that there is not enough cast iron
    evidence to show just how well childhood cholesterol
    levels predict adult levels to warrant universal screening
    of all children. In fact, studies show that quite a few chil-
    dren with high cholesterol levels will not have high
    enough levels as adults to qualify for individualized

treatment. The harm of universal screening, experts argue, is that it would single out lots of children for repeat testing and perhaps prompt unwarranted treatment and the overuse of cholesterol-lowering drugs.

Q What studies are you talking about?

A In one study published in 1990, researchers tested the cholesterol levels of 2,367 children, aged 8 to 18, for a period of 10 years. Fifty-seven per cent of the girls and 30 per cent of the boys had been identified as having levels in the danger zone. But when the researchers looked at lipid tests on these same individuals 20 to 30 years later, only a quarter of the females and less than half of the males who were in the danger zone as children met the criteria for intervention as adults.

That's why, at this point, most doctors recommend screening only children who have a family history of premature heart disease or one parent with high cholesterol. Children who are overweight or have other risk factors may also be screened. Of course, selective screening means that some children at risk will be overlooked because a parent's cholesterol level or family history is unknown. But in general, most experts agree on this: if your child does not have these risk factors or is not extremely obese or is not eating mainly a high-fat diet, you can relax about cholesterol screening.

Q I have high cholesterol. If my child's test reveals high levels, should I limit pizza and chips and go for low-fat foods?

A You would be on the right track to do so. If a child above the age of two has an elevated cholesterol level, the first strategy is to change the menu while maintaining a healthy weight and encouraging physical activity. A child in the high blood-cholesterol range who adopts a diet lower in cholesterol and saturated fat will have lower overall cholesterol and lower LDLs throughout childhood, and very probably lower cholesterol as an adult as well, thus making him less likely to develop heart disease. In one study, 484 children aged 12 to 18 substituted low-choles-terol/low-saturated fat foods for those in the typical 'afflu-ent' diet, and reduced their intake of saturated fat from 15 to 10 per cent of their calories. The results? Their choles-terol levels fell after less than three weeks on the diet.

As you plan meals, think low-fat rather than diet, which has come to be equated with deprivation. We talk more about the benefits of low-fat eating in Chapter 5.

Q Does a reduced-fat diet provide enough nutrients for my growing child?

A Yes. A child can get the necessary calories, protein, vita-mins and minerals for normal growth. In fact, low-fat diets offer more in the way of nutrients since they offer lots of fruits, vegetables and grains, along with low-fat dairy products, lean meat and fish. However, you might want to consult your doctor or a qualified dietitian to guide you in preparing a healthy menu.

Q   **How long should we use this diet?**

A   Give it at least three to six months. If after that time your
child's total and LDL cholesterol remain above 230
mg/dL and 160 mg/dL respectively, and she is of normal
development and school age, your doctor might recommend using a **bile acid binding resin** drug. This is particularly important if your child has a positive family history of
heart disease or a low HDL level.

Q   **Just what are these resin drugs?**

A   The typical bile acid drugs used for children are cholestyramine or **colestipol** (Colestid), orange-flavoured
powders that are mixed with juice and taken during
meals, starting with one scoop twice daily and gradually
increasing. Long-term studies show these drugs are relatively safe and effective in children, and have fewer side-
effects than cholesterol-lowering drugs because they are
not absorbed by the intestine. The most common side-
effects are constipation, nausea and bloating. Close
monitoring for growth and vitamin deficiencies is necessary, however, as these drugs may interfere with proper
absorption of normal fats and fat-soluble vitamins and
folic acid. We discuss these drugs in detail in Chapter 6.

PEOPLE WITH INHERITED CHOLESTEROL PROBLEMS

Q If my mother or father is being treated for high blood cholesterol, does this mean I might have the same problem?

A You might. High cholesterol can be due to excess weight and other factors or it can be due to an inherited lipid abnormality. Among children screened because of premature heart disease in a parent or grandparent, approximately one-third have some form of lipid abnormality. The most common form of inherited high cholesterol passed by genes is **familial hypercholesterolaemia** (FH). This is caused by a defect in LDL receptors, the portals on membranes which allow cholesterol to move in and out of the cells. When **LDL receptors** are defective, cholesterol can't be adequately removed from the cells, so it accumulates and deposits in the arteries.

Q What are my chances of having FH? And if I have it, what can I expect?

A FH affects 1 in 500 people. If either your mother or father has FH, you have a 50 per cent chance of developing heart disease by the age of 40 if you're male or by the age of 50 if you're female. People who have inherited FH from both parents, which occurs in one in a million cases, develop heart disease before the age of 20 and have few, if any, functioning LDL receptors.

Q   **Are there any clues to tell who might have FH?**
A   The biggest clue is if either parent or a grandparent had a heart attack before the age of 60. Another clue is if your total cholesterol level is above 300 to 400 mg/dL, or your LDL level is well above 200 mg/dL. People who have inherited the FH gene from both parents have total cholesterol levels that top 600 to 1,000 mg/dL.

Q   **How about any visible clues of an inherited disorder?**
A   People with FH may have raised yellowish bumps, called **xanthomas**, which are fatty deposits of cholesterol which settle in the tendons of the knees, elbows or knuckles. Xanthomas usually show up in a person's twenties or thirties, but can appear in younger children, who may also have an opaque ring around the periphery of the cornea of their eyes.

Q   **What about tests which can show me for sure if I have FH?**
A   The positive test for FH shows that LDL receptors are defective and involves extracting cells from skin tissue and growing them in a culture. Your doctor may refer you to a lipid specialist who can perform this test. In the near future, tests may be available which help to identify genetic blood markers called **apolipoproteins**. These are the protein components of lipoproteins and seem to affect the clearance of cholesterol in people with inherited disorders, according to preliminary results from the Framingham Study.

Q   I have FH and my daughter (whose cholesterol is normal) is pregnant with her first child. How can we tell if my problem has passed on to the baby?

A   In familial hypercholesterolaemia babies, LDL levels in blood from the umbilical cord at birth measure twice as high as levels found in normal babies. A blood sample can then be taken after the age of one. The results will help you to get started early at controlling cholesterol so you can retard development of advanced atherosclerosis.

Q   My 48-year-old brother survived a heart attack and keeps nagging me to get my triglycerides checked, as I could be next. I'm in my mid-thirties. What is he talking about?

A   Besides inheriting high levels of cholesterol, people who develop heart disease before the age of 55 sometimes also inherit high triglyceride levels, which points to a condition known as **familial combined hyperlipidaemia** (FCH). Half of the people who have a first-degree relative – mother, father, sibling – with FCH also develop FCH. So if your HDL is too low, your LDL too high and your triglyceride level is also high (250 to 500 or above), you have probably inherited the FCH gene. And it may have passed to your offspring, so get your children's triglycerides checked.

Q   If I have an inherited high-cholesterol problem, am I doomed to a heart attack or stroke?

A   No. While you are more likely to have premature heart disease than someone without a family history of FH, you can control your cholesterol and reduce your odds of early heart attack by sticking to a low-cholesterol, low-fat diet. Adopting such a diet helps to increase the number of LDL receptors, which in turn leads to a decrease in LDL in the blood. Monitoring your cholesterol will be a lifelong process, however, and you'll also need to control high blood pressure, avoid smoking and shed excess weight so that you're no more than 20 pounds over your ideal weight.

Q   **When is drug treatment called for?**

A   That depends on how high your cholesterol level is, how old you are, and other risk factors. If your cholesterol is 600 mg/dL and you're 15 years old, it's best to get your cholesterol down as quickly as possible using medication. But if it's 280 mg/dL, it's better to start with dietary measures and wait until the age of 20 or 25 to start drugs.

For adults with cholesterol levels in the 500 mg/dL range, dietary methods can be started. If these do not work after a fair trial, drugs such as bile acid binding resins will remove LDL cholesterol and lower total cholesterol.

OLDER PEOPLE AND CHOLESTEROL

Q Let's say I'm over 70. Will there ever be an age when I can stop worrying about cholesterol and eat what I want?

A We don't yet know for certain. However, there is intriguing evidence from a Yale University study (published in the *Journal of the American Medical Association*) showing that cholesterol may not be as important a risk factor for older people as it is for the middle-aged.

For four years, Yale researchers followed up 1,000 people past 70, with an average age of 79. Their findings: neither high total cholesterol nor low HDLs appeared to increase the risk of dying of heart attack.

Q Does this mean that after the age of 70 I can forget about the cholesterol check?

A Let's put it this way: according to some reports, there is a push to have elderly people routinely screened for high cholesterol as part of an effort to counter the growing burden of the consequences of heart disease. But the Yale researchers believe this is unwarranted. In their view, until there's good evidence to show that benefits of screening and treatment outweigh harm for the elderly, people of 65 and older without heart disease should not be routinely screened. Nor should they be treated with drugs, which can have more serious side-effects in the elderly. Perhaps their most emphatic point is that the benefits of cholesterol-lowering treatment based on tests done on middle-aged people cannot and should not be applied to elderly people.

Q **Is this no-screening/no-treatment advice for pensioners generally accepted among heart experts?**

A Far from it. This opinion has been soundly challenged by many leading heart experts, who believe that screening and preventative cholesterol-lowering methods can help the elderly avoid debilitating heart attacks and strokes and perhaps keep them out of nursing homes. Many will make the point that as people get older, the risk of heart disease increases. A heart attack or a stroke may not kill you but they can deprive you of your independence and seriously damage your quality of life.

Q **So this group says that if I want to hang on to my health I should watch my cholesterol, no matter how old I get?**

A Yes. In the view of many, even if you are healthy at the age of 60, 70 or 80 but indulge in artery-clogging foods, for example, you are courting a catastrophe such as a heart attack or stroke, which could be devastating to your lifestyle. Evidence is strong that lowering your lipid levels also reduces vascular disease. Just how much you need to lower it and by what method, however, depends on the extent of vascular disease.

Q **How do you check that?**

A You can have a **carotid ultrasound test**.

Q   **What does that do, exactly?**

A   It measures the extent of **calcification** (hardening) in the arteries. It's more complicated than a blood test, but could be justified if there is a risk of your needing bypass or other surgery, or of the possibility of debilitation. If you have little vascular damage but your cholesterol is raised, watching what you eat and being active are prudent strategies and work effectively in the majority of people. Higher cholesterol or more extensive vascular disease may require cholesterol-lowering drugs, which seem to be well-tolerated by older people.

Q   **Does 'watching what I eat' mean skipping steak and homemade pie?**

A   Based on evidence to date, the best advice for older people may be to take a moderate approach to meals. The Yale researchers believe that overemphasizing a low-fat, low-cholesterol diet when combined with a limited income could disrupt an older person's nutritional intake and interfere with the enjoyment of eating, an important pleasurable activity. So if you aim to eat mainly foods low in saturated fat, you can probably keep the occasional steak, lobster, cheese cake and other tasty fare on your menu.

PEOPLE WITH TOO-LOW CHOLESTEROL

Q   You mentioned in Chapter 2 that very low cholesterol has been associated with some health problems. Can you tell me more about this?

A   As we said, a number of studies have found that men with very low cholesterol – usually 160 mg/dL or below – were more likely than men with normal cholesterol levels to die of causes other than heart disease.

Q   What about women with low cholesterol? Any potentially negative connection there?

A   Apparently not. These studies involved mostly men, and the link seems to hold only for men.

Q   Were these studies of men with naturally low cholesterol or of people being treated to lower their cholesterol?

A   Both. In the treatment studies, however, only those using cholesterol-lowering drugs, not those using diet and lifestyle changes (such as stopping smoking), were more likely to die of an illness unrelated to heart disease.

Q   And what were these men dying of?

A   A variety of causes, including some types of cancer, lung or digestive diseases, gallbladder problems, accidents or suicides and, in a few cases, haemorrhagic stroke (cerebral haemorrhage).

Q   **How are these illnesses associated with low cholesterol?**
A   The fact is that nobody knows for sure. We know that
    once cholesterol gets below a certain level there is an
    increased death rate, but, in spite of research into the
    possible causes, just why this happens remains obscure.

Q   **Well, how do experts think they might be related?**
A   There are lots of possible explanations. One is that
    cholesterol is lowered by some diseases themselves.
    People with chronic lung disease often lose weight and
    so may lower their cholesterol. People with liver disease
    have reduced production of cholesterol in their livers.
    And people with digestive problems might not absorb
    fats properly.

    In fact, there's some evidence to show that cancer
    causes blood-cholesterol levels to drop. Some investiga-
    tors have reported that, as a tumour grows, the cells
    actively take up LDL cholesterol, causing blood levels of
    LDL to drop. And research also shows that people who
    go into remission as a result of chemotherapy have a
    return to normal blood-cholesterol levels.

Q   **Well, that all makes sense. Why isn't that explanation
    accepted as the cause?**
A   Because when these analyses exclude the men who died
    within five or so years after the study ended, which
    presumably would eliminate most of those who had some
    kind of disease at the time of the study, the results remain
    the same: Men with very low cholesterol are still more
    likely to die prematurely than people with normal levels.

Q   **What about alcohol abuse? Couldn't it be causing both health problems and low cholesterol?**

A   Yes. The alcohol/low-cholesterol connection is this: in heavy drinkers, alcohol can damage the liver, hampering its cholesterol-making capacity and resulting in lower blood-cholesterol levels. In fact, doctors who do post-mortems say that people who die of cirrhosis of the liver often have remarkably clean arteries.

But the association seems to be weak, since cholesterol drops only when someone has severe liver disease, and the association remains even when people with severe liver disease are excluded.

Q   **What about the side-effects of cholesterol-lowering drugs? Could they be causing the increase in deaths?**

A   In some cases, yes. Both gemfibrozil and clofibrate, drugs we talk more about in Chapter 6, have been implicated in some deaths, especially those involving liver and gall-bladder disease.

Q   **Any other explanations?**

A   Some researchers speculate that, since cholesterol is a vital part of cell membranes and hormones in the body, too-low levels could cause a wide variety of diseases and dysfunction.

Q   **Such as?**

A   Everything from cancer and stroke to mood or behaviour problems which might lead to accidents or suicide.

Q   **Any proof that this is actually the case?**

A   Only a bit, and mostly in monkeys on cholesterol-lower-ing diets. For instance, monkeys fed a moderately low-fat diet have reduced levels of **serotonin**, a brain neuro-transmitter that helps to inhibit impulsive behaviour. These monkeys are also more aggressive than monkeys fed a high-fat diet, even though they get plenty to eat.

Q   **But do men who lower their cholesterol a lot get impulsive or aggressive?**

A   No one knows. It seem that no one has ever measured it. Research is, however, going on to study the effects of cholesterol-lowering on mood. These studies include measurements of mood-altering brain chemicals such as serotonin in men and women taking cholesterol-lowering drugs. It will also examine brain biochemistry in people with naturally low cholesterol levels.

Q   **So there's no proof that cholesterol-lowering drugs or a low-fat diet causes mood problems in humans?**

A   While there's some speculation that this could happen, there is as yet no proof. And there's some evidence to the contrary.

In one trial on children in which half the children were on a special cholesterol-lowering diet and the others on a normal diet, the researchers found no difference between the two groups in psychosocial development, depression or other things. Other doctors confirm that, even in patients whose total cholesterol is brought down to 160 mg/dL and their LDL down to about 100 mg/dL, they find no evidence of depression.

Q **So what does all this mean? Should I just not worry about my cholesterol and go have a cheeseburger?**

A No, it doesn't mean that at all. This is where it pays to weigh risks against benefits. Research clearly shows that in people with the highest risk – those who already have signs of coronary heart disease – the benefits of lowering cholesterol outweigh any possible risks. Experts say that it would be irresponsible to tell people in this category not to do everything they can – diet, and drugs, if necessary – to reduce their cholesterol levels into a low-risk range. All the doctors we talked with agree this is sound advice.

Q **But what if I simply have high, or borderline high, cholesterol but no signs of heart disease? What should I do then?**

A Here again, you have to consider your potential benefits and risks carefully and get your doctor's advice, experts say. Find out what risks for heart disease you can elimi-nate with no risk and little cost – give up smoking, lose weight and start exercising.

Changes in diet are now considered the preferred choice for lowering cholesterol for most people. Changing to a safe and appropriate diet has never had anything but beneficial side-effects – like preventing cancer, diabetes, obesity and high blood pressure.

If you have a serious inherited cholesterol disorder, however, you may benefit from taking drugs to reduce your cholesterol, even though you have no signs of heart disease.

Q Does this mean there is an ideal cholesterol range
A which you shouldn't try to go below?
As mentioned earlier, most problems seem to occur at cholesterol levels of 160 mg/dL or lower. This low level is achievable on either diet or drug therapy, or both. So you might want to aim for not much lower than that, with LDL levels of about 100 mg/dL.

CHAPTER FIVE

CHOLESTEROL-
AND TRIGLYCERIDE-
LOWERING DIETS

REVERSING CORONARY
ARTERY DISEASE

Q I know we'll be discussing the types of diet that help to prevent heart disease, but I'd like to know first – can you actually reverse atherosclerosis if your blood levels of cholesterol are low enough?

A Yes. A number of studies have found it is possible for some people to undo at least some of the artery-choking effects of years of burgers and chips.

Q What exactly do these studies show?

A One report looked at 11 studies, involving a total of 2,095 men and women. All 10 were randomized, controlled clinical trials using coronary **arteriography** (a test which can measure obstruction inside an artery) to assess the effects of lowering cholesterol. In other words, these studies were carefully designed and had an objective means of measuring results.

Q **So what did they find?**

A The researchers found that artery obstruction diminished in nearly one-third of those on an aggressive cholesterol-lowering treatment programme. Only one-tenth of people who received modest interventions (a moderately reduced-fat diet and, usually, bile acid binding resins, which we talk about in Chapter 6) had diminished obstructions.

And in the six studies that reported cardiovascular events, there were fewer heart attacks among the aggressively treated individuals.

Q **What does that mean – aggressive treatment? Were these studies lowering cholesterol a lot?**

A Yes. They reduced it further than is done in most studies, achieving, on average, a 28 per cent reduction in LDL cholesterol, an 11 per cent reduction in triglycerides and an 11 per cent increase in HDL cholesterol, compared with control groups, which lowered total blood cholesterol an average of 10 per cent.

Q **What does that mean in terms of actual cholesterol levels?**

A In these studies, the figures averaged out this way for the aggressively treated group: Triglycerides averaged 172 mg/dL to start; they dropped 11 per cent, to 153 mg/dL. Total cholesterol was 276 mg/dL; it dropped 26 per cent, to 205 mg/dL. LDL, at 196 mg/dL, dropped 36 per cent to 125 mg/dL. And HDL, initially at 42 mg/dL, rose 17 per cent to 49 mg/dL.

Q   But these figures aren't as low as the target goals cited earlier for people with heart disease. Why not?

A   That's true, they're not. Some doctors believe a large percentage drop in cholesterol helps to reverse the course of heart disease as much as reaching a particular target figure. And if these people could go even lower, perhaps they'd see even more reversal. One expert said: 'We look most at LDL cholesterol, and we like to see it below 100 mg/dL.' That's usually along with total cholesterol of 160 to 180 mg/dL and HDL levels above 30 mg/dL.

Q   Did these studies use drugs or diet?

A   Four of the studies used diet, exercise and the like; seven used single- and multiple-drug therapy combined with diet.

Q   Which worked better, drugs or diet?

A   Two of the non-drug studies worked better than any of the drug studies. Patients in both had about a 40 per cent greater rate of regression than those in a control group – that is, they were 40 per cent more likely to have shrinkage of artery blockages.

Q   What kinds of diets were used in these studies?

A   The diet used in these was mostly vegetarian, rich in vegetables, fruits, grains and beans, which are naturally low in fat and high in fibre. Total fat intake was cut to 10 per cent of calories. Foods of animal origin were limited to non-fat dairy products and egg whites and one serving of lean poultry or fish (no red meat) three times a week.

This diet had about 20 grams of fat for a 1,800-calorie-a-day total. Those taking part avoided every known booster of blood cholesterol – too much total fat, saturated fat, **trans fatty acids** and dietary cholesterol. (We discuss these dietary components later in this chapter.) They also ate lots of soluble fibre, which also helps to reduce cholesterol. And lots of vitamin E, vitamin C and **beta-carotene**, a vitamin A precursor. All three of these nutrients, especially vitamin E, appear to help stop the early stage of atherosclerosis mentioned in Chapter 1: the oxidation of LDL cholesterol.

Q   How long does it take to see results using such a diet?
A   Less time than you might think. Most studies saw plaque shrinkage in only two to four years – that's considered a relatively short period of time as far as arterial disease goes.

Q   How exactly do these fatty plaques shrink?
A   The details aren't entirely known, but only 'active' plaques – those that still contain macrophages and aren't completely covered with fibre and minerals – seem to be able to reverse. And once cholesterol levels get low enough in the blood, LDL cholesterol may move out of the plaque into an area of lower concentration, where, apparently, it is picked up by HDL and carried to the liver.

Q   How much shrinkage can you expect to see in these fatty plaques?
A   Studies show that, most of the time, they shrink just a bit – in most cases, less than 2 per cent.

Q   **Two per cent? That's not very much. Does it make any difference?**

A   For starters, it means the plaque isn't increasing in size by about 1.5 per cent, as it otherwise would do. And even with this small amount of shrinkage, there's still an improvement in symptoms – more than one might expect. That's apparently because the reduction in cholesterol levels also improves the function of endothelial cells – the cells lining the arteries.

Q   **What has that got to do with it?**

A   These cells do more than act as a tube for blood. They secrete biochemicals which play an important role in the health of the circulatory system. For one thing, they secrete chemicals that help blood vessels relax. This can help to protect against the **vasospasms** which can cause angina, or chest pains caused by a lack of oxygen to the heart.

Endothelial cells also secrete chemicals which cut down platelet stickiness and so reduce the tendency for clotting at the site of a plaque. It is the clotting of blood on top of a plaque that leads to the complete blockage of an artery – such as a branch of a coronary artery. And it is the action of the platelets that initiates the clotting. So these functions are very important when it comes to preventing heart attacks.

Q   **Did any of these studies include people who had had bypass surgery?**

A   Yes. The Cholesterol-lowering and Atherosclerosis

Study included men who had had bypass surgery. Half the men took two cholesterol-lowering drugs, colestipol and nicotinic acid (see *Chapter 6*). The other half took a placebo. The men's progress was followed up for a total of four years.

Q So what happened? Did the drugs help to keep the bypass surgery grafts open?

A In a word, yes. And it was most apparent in the fourth year of the study that the drugs were helpful. Arteriograms done then showed non-progression of fatty plaques in 52 per cent of men taking the two drugs, compared with only 15 per cent of men in the placebo group. And regression was 18 per cent in the treated group, compared with 6 per cent in those taking the placebo.

People in the treatment group were also less likely to have new fatty plaques in the non-grafted, or 'native' arteries. Fourteen per cent had new plaques, compared with 40 per cent in the placebo group. And in their bypass grafts, new plaques occurred in only 14 per cent, versus 38 per cent in the placebo group.

Q That's important, isn't it? I've heard that bypasses can clog up quite quickly.

A They can. The rate of progression of fatty plaques is reported to be three to six times greater in grafted than in non-grafted vessels. Without intervention to lower cholesterol, 45 per cent of grafts are seriously clogged up five years after bypass surgery.

Q How much of a role does diet really play in high cholesterol? Or are bad genes to blame?

A It's true that some people have inherited disorders which keep their cholesterol or triglyceride levels high despite dietary measures. And some people can eat just about anything they want and never have a problem with high cholesterol. But most people fall somewhere in between.

The results of trials of low-fat, low-cholesterol diets are variable. Some people will drop their cholesterol 100 mg/dL or more on such a diet, others' levels hardly change at all. We don't know exactly how many people are truly resistant to dietary changes. Most studies simply look at average declines in cholesterol, and researchers assume that the people who don't respond are being 'non-compliant' – not following the diet.

One type of study – metabolic ward studies, where people are, basically, paid captives whose every bite is controlled – shows that it is indeed rare for a person not to respond at all to diet. The only way to know how much you'll respond to a diet – and if you are truly diet-resistant – is to try a particular diet and see if it lowers your cholesterol. If you already have heart disease, a low-fat diet may also reduce your symptoms of chest pain, fatigue and so forth.

Q So most people can reduce their cholesterol with diet?

A Yes. Most doctors today believe that too much fat in the diet, especially saturated fat, plays a major role in raising cholesterol levels. They point to the fact that in countries where a low-saturated-fat diet is the norm, such as the traditional rice-and-fish Japanese menu, cholesterol levels average 160 mg/dL or lower. But when these people switch to a high-fat European or American diet, their cholesterol levels rise, along with their risk of heart disease.

Doctors also cite the fact that most people, if they are willing to work at it, can lower their cholesterol on a sufficiently low-fat diet and, in some cases, can even slightly shrink artery blockages.

Q   **So is that what causes high blood cholesterol? A high-fat diet?**

A   It's certainly one major reason. We all need some fat in our diets. But we need only enough to supply our bodies with adequate amounts of two essential fatty acids, **linoleic** and **linolenic** acid. It's possible to get this amount by eating 15 to 25 grams of the kind of fat that characterizes the typical Western diet. However, the best sources are vegetable oils – rapeseed (**canola oil**), safflower, corn, soybean and cottonseed.

But most people get 80 to 100 grams of fat a day. That's the problem – too much fat, especially saturated fats.

Some doctors think a high saturated-fat diet puts everyone at risk of coronary artery disease, and to some extent statistics back them up. If you don't die of cancer, the chances are high that you'll die of a heart attack, a stroke or some other problem associated with atherosclerosis.

Q **But don't other things besides a high-fat diet raise cholesterol?**

A Yes. Stress can raise cholesterol levels, as can disorders of the liver, gallbladder or thyroid. And as mentioned earlier, high cholesterol is only one of numerous risk factors for heart disease. Since most people in developed countries have at least borderline high cholesterol – 200 to 249 mg/dL – these other risk factors play an important role in determining who is most at risk.

But since high cholesterol seems so closely linked with a high-fat diet, which can easily enough be pared down, and since a high-fat diet is associated with another big killer, cancer, a lot of the emphasis these days is on cutting out fat, especially saturated fats and **hydrogenated fats**, which we'll explain shortly.

Q **Exactly what kind of diet is recommended to reduce cholesterol?**

A These days there are a number of diets; some cut fat only a bit, to just under 30 per cent of calories, and are recommended for anyone wanting a healthy diet, high cholesterol or not. Others slash fat to the bone, to 10 per cent or less of calories, and are geared towards people who already have blocked arteries or very high cholesterol. In between are moderately reduced-fat diets, with 15 to 25 per cent of one's calories coming in the form of fat.

And some doctors recommend a Mediterranean-style diet, which has 25 to 30 per cent total fat – mostly from a **monounsaturated fat**, olive oil – but which is low in saturated fats.

SATURATED FATS

Q Before we go any further, explain these fats to me.
   What exactly are saturated fats?

A Saturated fats are solid at room temperature. They are
   the main component of the white marbling in meats, of
   the visible fat around meat, of butter and cheese and of
   whole milk and ice cream. Saturated fats are also plenti-
   ful in coconut oil, palm kernel oil and palm oil – three
   plant oils widely used in commercial baked goods such as
   biscuits and cakes.

Q But why are they called saturated?

A This is a chemical term referring to the structure of the
   three fatty acids joined to the glycerol backbone in fats
   (triglycerides). Carbon atoms (the stuff of all organic
   matter) can link to hydrogen atoms and many other
   atoms, as well as to each other. When all four linkages of
   a carbon atom are taken up by single links to other
   atoms, the molecule is said to be saturated. If some have
   more than one link (are doubled or trebled) the molecule is said to be unsaturated. Unsaturated linkages can
   readily allow other atoms to join on. Saturated linkages
   are more stable.

Q Why are saturated fats supposed to be so bad for you?

A Most saturated fats – although there are exceptions –
   raise blood levels of LDL cholesterol. They do this,
   apparently, by increasing cholesterol production in the
   body and by inhibiting the uptake of LDL cholesterol by

cells. Cells can't take in cholesterol that is circulating in the blood as easily when you're eating a high saturated-fat diet as they can when saturated-fat intake is low.

Q   **Do most people eat a lot of saturated fat?**

A   Certainly. The average person in Britain can really put it away. Most of us get about 14 per cent of our calories from saturated fat. Researchers have calculated that each percent of calories from saturated fat raises total cholesterol by approximately 2.3 mg/dL. In fact, saturated fats raise blood-cholesterol levels more than dietary cholesterol does. The yolk of eggs contain a large amount of cholesterol but it is known that some people can eat large numbers of eggs without greatly affecting the cholesterol levels in their bodies.

Q   **But I've heard saturated fat is not so bad. What's the truth about this?**

A   You may have heard about a component of saturated fat, called **stearic acid**, found in red meat and chocolate. Recent research suggests that stearic acid does not elevate LDL cholesterol. However, stearic acid is only one small fraction of the fatty acids found in saturated fats.

Q   **What is the main fatty acid in saturated fats?**

A   It's a component called palmitic acid, and it's the predominant saturated fat in red meat, chicken and butter fat, and even in certain vegetable fats and oils, such as palm, cottonseed and cocoa butter.

Q   **Does palmitic acid raise LDL cholesterol levels?**

A   Yes, definitely. And palmitic acid is the component of saturated fat people in Britain eat most. Most people get 8 to
10 per cent of their calories from palmitic acid, an amount
calculated to raise their cholesterol by 22 to 27 mg/dL.

TRANS FATTY ACIDS

Q   **What about fats in margarine and vegetable shorten-
ing? Aren't they solid at room temperature?**

A   These products contain hydrogenated vegetable oil.
Manufacturers have added hydrogen, which makes these
products harder and also helps to keep them from
becoming rancid. Hydrogenated vegetable oils contain
trans fatty acids.

Q   **Do trans fatty acids raise cholesterol levels?**

A   Yes. They act in ways similar to saturated fats.

About half a dozen studies have found that the
amount of trans fatty acids found in the typical Western
diet – 8 to 15 grams a day – can raise LDL cholesterol
levels as much as saturated fats do. One study also found
that about twice that amount – 30 grams a day –
lowered HDL cholesterol by about 13 per cent, which
translates into a 26 per cent increase in risk for heart
disease.

A study by Harvard University researchers, for
instance, found women with the highest intake of trans
fatty acids (about 6 grams a day) were 50 per cent more

likely to develop heart disease than those who took in less than half as much. They also found that those who ate four or more teaspoons a day of margarine raised their risks of heart problems by 66 per cent, compared with those who ate less than one teaspoon a month. The researchers saw no such risk from butter.

Another study compared how trans fatty acids compared with saturated fats, such as those found in butter. Considering LDL alone, the study estimated that 1 gram of trans fat has 0.7 times the cholesterol-raising capacity of the same amount of saturated fat. Taking the drop in HDL levels into account would boost that number to 1.3. However, many researchers believe that most people don't eat enough trans fatty acids to affect their HDL levels.

Q So what should I do? Not eat margarine? Eat butter instead?

A If you must have some kind of spread on bread, stick to soft-spread margarines, which have fewer trans fatty acids per gram than ordinary margarines. Look for those that list water or a liquid vegetable oil as the first ingredient. If you've been melting margarine to use in cooking, switch to olive or rapeseed oil instead.

If you prefer butter to margarine and your overall risk of heart disease is low, you can use butter sparingly without feeling guilty.

Q How much trans fatty acid can I safely eat?

A Researchers are now saying that you should lump trans

fatty acids with saturated fats. That means you shouldn't be getting more than 10 per cent of your calories from saturated fats and trans fatty acids combined – from about 18 to 26 grams a day for most people.

Margarine, fried fast foods and packaged baked goods are the main sources of trans fatty acids for most people in Britain. A fried fish sandwich has 8.2 grams; a fried fruit pie, 5.9 grams; a plain doughnut, 3.2 grams; a small order of chips, 3.6 grams; a tablespoon of ordinary margarine, 3.1; two small sweet biscuits, 1.7.

Baked goods marketed as 'made with all vegetable oils' may be high in trans fatty acids. If so, you will see hydrogenated or partially hydrogenated vegetable oil as one of the first three ingredients on their labels.

POLYUNSATURATED FATS

Q   **What are polyunsaturated fats?**
A   Polyunsaturated fats are liquid at room temperature and are the predominant fat in common vegetable oils, such as corn, safflower, sunflower, cottonseed, soybean and walnut oils.

One reason for the corn-oil craze back in the 1970s was that some studies suggested that unsaturated fats such as the 'polys' can actually reduce total cholesterol. In fact, however, research now suggests that, while polyunsaturated fats do not raise harmful LDL cholesterol, they do lower helpful HDL cholesterol. This is hardly a desirable result. And in animals, at least, diets high in polyunsaturated fats may increase the risk of cancer.

These fats are also easily oxidized. That means that, in your body, incorporated into LDL they react with oxygen in a chemical reaction that's identical to butter becoming rancid. As we explained in Chapter I, oxidation of LDL cholesterol is thought to be one of the initial stages of fatty plaque development in arteries. So it's good to keep your intake of these fats fairly low. We talk about the antioxidant properties of some vitamins, especially vitamin E, later in this chapter.

MONOUNSATURATED FATS

Q **What about the monounsaturated fats you mentioned earlier?**

A Monounsaturated fats are also liquid at room temperature. Olive oil is 77 per cent monounsaturated fat. Rapeseed (canola) oil is 58 per cent monounsaturated. Peanut oil contains some monounsaturated fat.

Q **I've heard that olive oil is supposed to be good to use if you are concerned about high cholesterol. Is it?**

A It does seem to be. In studies, switching from saturated to monounsaturated fats, such as olive oil, made LDL cholesterol drop without also dropping HDL cholesterol. Studies from French researchers suggest that a diet rich in olive oil changes the structure of HDL, increasing its capacity to transport LDL cholesterol to the liver for disposal.

Other studies suggest that olive oil is less prone to oxidation than polyunsaturated fat. In 'olive-oil belt' countries – Greece and Italy, for instance – people eat a diet that's fairly high in monounsaturated fats but low in saturated fats. And their risk of heart disease is a fraction of that in Britain. Olive oil contains more heart-protective vitamin E than other vegetable oils, which may be one reason for its apparent heart-healthy benefits.

DIETARY CHOLESTEROL

Q   You haven't mentioned anything about dietary cholesterol. Isn't it important to limit the amount of cholesterol you eat, too?

A   That used to be the received wisdom, but it's now open to debate. Most authorities still agree, however, that too much dietary cholesterol does raise your blood level of cholesterol, and recommend you get no more than 300 mg of cholesterol a day from foods. (That comes to no more than three to four large eggs a week.) On an average day, a man consumes about 450 mg and a woman about 320 mg of cholesterol.

Q   Why is this open to debate? Doesn't eating too much cholesterol raise your cholesterol?

A   Not for everybody and, apparently, not even for most people, once total fat and saturated fat are reduced. Studies indicate that about one person in three has a significant drop in blood cholesterol if they lower cholesterol in the diet. Such people would benefit by reducing their dietary intake of cholesterol by 200 mg or more.

There's also a small group that can eat practically unlimited amounts of cholesterol a day with no change in blood cholesterol. And then there's a large middle group of people who have minor responses to dietary cholesterol.

Q **How will I know if I should cut back?**
A If your total, HDL and LDL cholesterol are all within safe ranges, then you're probably safe to go on eating whatever cholesterol you've been eating. However, if your cholesterol is high, you'll want to keep your egg intake down to three to four a week, since eggs contain saturated fat in addition to cholesterol.

Q **How much cholesterol actually is in an egg?**
A An egg yolk from one large egg contains a little more than 200 mg of cholesterol and about 5.1 grams of fat; 1.6 grams of it is saturated fat. Many baked goods contain egg yolks, unless the label says they are cholesterol-free.

Q **I've heard liver contains a lot of cholesterol. Is it OK to eat?**
A If your cholesterol is normal, there's no reason not to have a serving of liver now and then, since liver is packed with nutrients, such as vitamins B_{12} and A. It's true that liver and other organ meats, such as sweetbreads

(thymus or pancreas), brain and heart, are loaded with cholesterol. Three ounces of beef liver yield 331 mg of cholesterol. That same serving contains only 1.6 grams of saturated fat, but if your cholesterol is high, you're better off avoiding it.

FISH AND SHELLFISH

Q **What about prawns? I've heard they're not so bad to eat.**

A Certain shellfish, such as prawns and crayfish, are higher in cholesterol than most other types of fish and seafood. But they're lower in total fat and saturated fat than most meats and poultry. Three ounces of prawns have 166 mg of cholesterol, but only 0.25 mg of saturated fat. So you're better off eating prawns than those other foods. Just make sure you eat them steamed, not fried, which adds lots of fat.

Q **What about other seafoods?**

A A research study found that men who substituted oysters, crab, lobster, clams, mussels or scallops for cheese, meat or eggs had a reduction in LDL cholesterol and an increase in HDL cholesterol. Prawns and squid didn't improve cholesterol levels, but they didn't harm them, either.

Q **Isn't there some sort of oil in fish that's supposed to be good for your heart?**

A Yes. Some fatty fish such as salmon, mackerel, tuna and

some shellfish contain **omega-3 fatty acids**. Smaller amounts are also found in whole grains, beans, seaweed and soybean products. And purslane, a fleshy, low-growing weed sometimes used in salads, contains high amounts of omega-3 fatty acid.

These fats are polyunsaturated but their chemical structure is different from other polyunsaturated fats.

Q   **What do omega-3 fatty acids do for cholesterol levels?**
A   They don't seem to have any effect at all on cholesterol, but they do lower triglycerides in some people. That is not apparently, however, their main benefit when it comes to preventing heart disease. The biggest benefit of fish oils may come from their ability to reduce a process called **platelet aggregation**, an important part of blood clotting in which platelets stick together to form a mass that is the beginning of a blood clot. A diet rich in fish oils helps to keep platelets from sticking together and from sticking to artery walls. (Aspirin has the same effect.) This means blood clots are less likely to form on top of cholesterol deposits (plaques).

Fish oils also dampen the body's inflammatory response, which may play a role in the early development of atherosclerosis.

Q   **Does this mean I should eat more fish?**
A   Certainly, substitute fish for some of the beef or chicken you are eating. Some experts recommend up to three fish meals a week. However, since even fish contains some saturated fat, if you're going super-low-fat, you'll

want to stick mostly with the vegetable sources of omega-3 fatty acids – seaweeds, soybeans and purslane.

Q **What about fish-oil capsules?**

A You're better off eating fish. Three ounces of mackerel, tuna or salmon offer 2,500 mg of omega-3 fatty acids, while a typical omega-3 capsule contains only 300 mg. These capsules are made up mostly of other fats.

SUGAR AND ALCOHOL

Q **You've talked about foods that affect cholesterol levels. Are there any foods that affect triglyceride levels?**

A Alcohol and simple carbohydrates, such as sugar, raise triglyceride levels directly through their effect on the liver. They cause the liver to produce VLDL (very low-density lipoprotein) cholesterol, which then breaks down to form triglycerides and LDL cholesterol.

Q **Alcohol raises triglyceride levels? But I've heard wine is supposed to be good for your heart. Is it?**

A Studies show that moderate drinking – one drink a day for women, two for men – is associated with a reduced risk of heart attacks. In fact, the reduction in risk is comparable to the protection conferred by taking low-dose aspirin, stopping smoking, exercising or losing weight.

Q **How does alcohol work?**

A One or two drinks a day increase HDL cholesterol 5 to

10 mg/dL. Alcohol also reduces the tendency for blood clotting, a factor in clogged arteries. And the substances that give red wine and grape juice their deep rich colour may also inhibit the oxidation of LDL cholesterol in artery walls.

Q But should I avoid alcohol if my triglyceride levels are
A high?

Yes. In that case, the potential negative effects – higher-than-ever triglyceride levels – outweigh any potential benefits.

Q Don't fats also raise triglyceride levels?
A Dietary fats *are* triglycerides, so they will certainly raise triglyceride levels immediately after a meal, but this triglyceride is a special, temporary form. It is transported in **chylomicrons**, tiny spheres of fat that go directly from the intestines to the liver. Chylomicrons are thought to have no direct effect on the development of atherosclerosis.

One reason triglyceride levels sometimes rise when people go on low-fat diets is that they are substituting carbohydrates and sugar for fat. Some people with high triglyceride levels, and especially those with diabetes, actually do better in terms of cholesterol and blood-sugar control if they eat a diet that contains a bit more monounsaturated fat and fewer carbohydrates and sugar.

WHEN TO GO LOW-FAT

Q   **How high does someone's cholesterol need to be for a doctor to recommend a low-fat diet?**

A   Here are some guidelines for starting a low-fat diet:

- If you haven't got heart disease and have fewer than two of the risk factors listed in Table B (*page 42*), such as smoking or high blood pressure, it's recommended you start dietary therapy if your LDL cholesterol is more than 160 mg/dL. Your goal should be to keep your LDL cholesterol below 160 mg/dL and your total cholesterol lower than 240 mg/dL.

- If you haven't got heart disease but have two or more risk factors, it's recommended you start dietary therapy if your LDL cholesterol is more than 130 mg/dL. Your goal is to keep your LDL cholesterol under 130 mg/dL and your total cholesterol under 200 mg/dL.

- If you have heart disease, dietary intervention should start when LDL cholesterol is higher than 100 mg/dL; the goal is to keep LDL under 100 mg/dL and total cholesterol at 160 mg/dL or less.

Q   **What kinds of dietary recommendations are made?**

A   The experts advise that doctors should start their patients on one of two diets – known as Step I and Step II diets.

The Step I Diet calls for 30 per cent or less of calories from fat, with 8 to 10 per cent of calories from saturated fat and 300 mg or less of cholesterol a day. Your doctor may suggest this diet to ease you into a lower-fat diet, especially if your current diet is very high in fat.

Q   **How does the Step I diet differ from what most people eat?**
A   Studies show that a typical British diet has 40 per cent of calories from fat, with 13 to 14 per cent saturated, 14 per cent monounsaturated and 8 per cent polyunsaturated fats, and a cholesterol intake of 350 to 400 mg a day.

Q   **So what does the Step I diet look like on a plate?**
A   The Step I diet is not particularly stringent. It's the kind of diet most doctors these days encourage everyone to follow. For 1,800 calories a day, the amount most women eat, a Step I diet looks something like this:

Breakfast $^1/_2$ medium bread roll, I teaspoon low-fat cream cheese, I cup shredded wheat cereal, I small banana, I cup semi-skimmed milk, $^3/_4$ cup orange juice and a cup of coffee with 2 tablespoons semi-skimmed milk.

Lunch $^1/_2$ cup minestrone soup, I roast beef sandwich made with 2 slices of wholewheat bread, 3 ounces lean roast beef, $^3/_4$ ounce low-fat cheese, I leaf of lettuce, 3 slices of tomato and 2 teaspoons of low-fat mayonnaise, I medium apple and I cup of water.

Dinner   3 ounces salmon, I medium baked potato with I teaspoon soft-spread margarine, $^1/_2$

cup green beans with $^1/_2$ teaspoon soft-spread margarine, $^1/_2$ cup carrots with $^1/_2$ teaspoon soft-spread margarine, one medium white dinner roll with 1 teaspoon soft-spread margarine, $^1/_2$ cup semi-skimmed milk and a cup of unsweetened tea.

Snack   2 cups of popcorn with 1 teaspoon soft-spread margarine.

Q   **What kind of results can you expect to see on this sort of diet?**

A   A wide range – from 3 to 14 per cent cholesterol reduction – depending on your cholesterol level and your eating habits when you start the diet. The higher your blood-cholesterol level and the fattier your regular diet, the more of a drop you are likely see on a low-fat diet. Men eating an average British diet can expect a drop of 5 to 7 per cent in total cholesterol. Women may see slightly less of a drop.

The only way to find out for sure how you are going to respond is to try the diet. Incidentally, people who drop excess weight on a low-fat diet often have much better cholesterol-lowering results. We talk more about obesity and heart disease in Chapter 7.

Q   **How long do I need to be on this diet before I know if it is going to work?**

A   A minimum of three months. Then you'll have your blood level of cholesterol checked to see how much it has dropped.

Q **What happens if this diet doesn't do the trick for me?**

A The Step I diet has been criticized for not cutting fat enough to do much good. So it may not be restrictive enough for you.

If you're actually sticking to the diet – and any exercise and weight-loss recommendations your doctor has advised – and your cholesterol still hasn't dropped enough after three months, your doctor will most likely recommend a diet that is more restrictive in saturated fat – the Step II diet.

Q **How is it different from the Step I diet?**

A This diet reduces saturated fat to less than 7 per cent of calories, and cholesterol to less than 200 mg a day. But it allows more servings of vegetable fats and oils (poly- and monounsaturated fats), thereby keeping total calories from fat the same as for Step I – 30 per cent. Most of the reduction in saturated fat comes from smaller portions of meat and cheese, and having skimmed milk instead of semi-skimmed.

Q **So what does that look like on a plate?**

A For 1,800 calories a day, a Step II daily menu plan might look like this:

Breakfast ½ medium bread roll, 1 teaspoon jam, 1 cup shredded wheat cereal, 1 small banana, 1 cup skimmed milk, 1 cup orange juice and a cup of coffee with 2 tablespoons skimmed milk.

Lunch $^1/_2$ cup minestrone soup, I roast beef sand-
            wich made with 2 slices wholewheat bread, 2
            ounces lean roast beef, $^3/_4$ ounce low-fat
            cheese, I leaf lettuce, 3 slices of tomato and
            2 teaspoons soft-spread margarine, I
            medium apple and I cup of water.

Dinner   3 ounces flounder, I teaspoon vegetable oil,
            I medium baked potato with I teaspoon
            soft-spread margarine, $^1/_2$ cup green beans
            with $^1/_2$ teaspoon soft-spread margarine, $^1/_2$
            cup carrots with $^1/_2$ teaspoon soft-spread
            margarine, one medium white dinner roll
            with I teaspoon soft-spread margarine, $^1/_2$
            cup low-fat frozen yoghurt and a cup of
            unsweetened tea.

Snack   3 cups of popcorn with 2 teaspoons soft-
            spread margarine.

Q   **What kind of results can you expect to see on the Step
    II diet?**

A   Another 3 to 7 per cent reduction in total cholesterol,
    which, added to the 3 to 14 per cent achieved by the
    Step I diet, results in a total of 6 to 20 per cent.

Q   **How long a time are people supposed to give this diet?**

A   A minimum of three months, but some doctors say it
    takes people longer than that really to learn how to
    follow such a diet. They recommend giving it a year, if
    possible, before considering the use of drugs.

Q What's the best way to ensure that such a diet will work for me?

A First, make quite sure that you are fully aware of the implications of *not* sticking to the diet. The diet will work for you, all right; the real problem is, will you work at sticking to the diet? Most experts are rather cynical about this. But if you really understand that this is your principal chance of ensuring a long, healthy life and avoiding disasters such as heart attacks or strokes, with all the attendant loss of quality of life, you may be able to prove the experts wrong.

Q Can my doctor refer me to a dietitian?

A He or she could do, but this is not going to help if you are not serious about your dieting. It's really up to you. A dietitian could certainly give you lots of excellent advice; the question is whether you are going to comply with it. In the US, people rely heavily on dietitians and spend a lot of money consulting them. But the proof of the pudding is, in this case, in the *not* eating, and there is little indication that Americans, as a whole, have benefited from expert dietetic advice.

VITAMINS AND HEART DISEASE

Q Can't certain vitamins help to prevent heart disease?

A Apparently so. As already mentioned, vitamins E and C and beta-carotene all appear to help reduce the risk of heart disease. All three function as antioxidants. They help to protect LDL cholesterol from oxidation – reacting with oxygen – a first step in the process of atherosclerosis, as discussed in Chapter 1. Vitamin E does the job directly, by entering the artery wall in the same lipoprotein particles that carry LDL cholesterol. The role of beta-carotene is less well understood; it may also enter the arterial wall to provide protection against oxidation. The main role of vitamin C in all this is apparently to protect vitamin E so it can keep on protecting against the LDL cholesterol. C and E act co-operatively to provide an excellent antioxidant effect.

Q But do these vitamins actually lower cholesterol?
A So far only one, vitamin C, seems to influence cholesterol levels. Researchers have found that large doses of vitamin C lower LDL and raise HDL levels. They found that women's HDL peaked when vitamin C in their blood reached 1 mg/dL. For men, HDL continued to rise parallel with vitamin C, while the LDL cholesterol dropped significantly.

For women, the amount needed to reach that blood concentration was about 90 mg – the amount in $^{1}/_{3}$ pint of orange juice. Men reached the same concentration when they had consumed about 150 mg. Since vitamin C levels drop quickly after a large dose, most experts suggest you take at least two doses a day.

It's possible to get enough vitamin C and beta-carotene in your diet by eating lots of fruits and vegetables, especially citrus fruits and dark leafy greens. To get protective amounts of vitamin E – at least 400 IU (international units) a day, according to one study — requires supplements.

Q **Do any other vitamins or minerals affect cholesterol or triglycerides?**

A We talk about the B vitamin niacin, which is often used in large doses to lower cholesterol, in Chapter 6. The form of niacin that's actually used is nicotinic acid.

One other nutrient deserves mention here — chromium. Chromium deficiency seems to play a role in the development of atherosclerosis. Several studies have shown that one form of this trace mineral, chromium picolinate, may help to reduce high LDL cholesterol and triglyceride levels and raise HDL levels. And it seems especially helpful to people with diabetes.

In one study, for instance, moderately obese non-insulin-dependent diabetics who took 200 micrograms (mcg) of chromium picolinate every day for two months experienced a 17.4 per cent drop in triglyceride levels. There was no change while they were taking a placebo.

Q **Can I get that much chromium from foods?**

A It's not likely. Most diets don't contain enough chromium. Brewer's yeast, wheat germ, broccoli, cheese and prunes are good sources, but you may need to take supplements to reach cholesterol-lowering amounts. Some doctors recommend up to 200 mcg three times a day to their patients with diabetes and high triglycerides. However, these high doses should never be taken without medical supervision. Although no toxicity has been reported in amounts up to 600 mcg a day, chromium can be toxic.

Q   **What about the B vitamin folic acid? I've read that it's supposed to help prevent heart disease. Does it?**

A   Apparently so. Low levels of folic acid increase blood levels of homocysteine, an amino acid that may damage the endothelial cells lining the artery walls, making it easier for LDL cholesterol to deposit there. Folic acid does not affect blood-cholesterol levels, however.

To keep homocysteine levels low, researchers suggest you get 400 mcg a day of folic acid. Most people get about half that amount in a normal daily diet. To reach 400 mcg, include orange juice (one cup has 110 mcg), leafy greens (one cup of raw spinach has 130 mcg) and vitamin supplements or folate-fortified breakfast cereals in your daily diet.

CHAPTER SIX

CHOLESTEROL-
AND TRIGLYCERIDE-
LOWERING DRUGS

GUIDELINES FOR USING
CHOLESTEROL-LOWERING DRUGS

Q When are drugs used to lower cholesterol or triglyceride levels?

A Drugs are meant to be used only in addition to lifestyle measures, such as eating a low-fat diet, stopping smoking, losing weight and exercising. That's true even for people who need drugs from the start because of high initial cholesterol or triglyceride levels. It's also true for people with moderately high levels who have tried and failed to lower their cholesterol with changes in lifestyle.

Q But diets are hard to stick to, and not everyone can manage to amend their lifestyles. Why can't people just take drugs?

A Because all the drugs used to lower cholesterol and triglycerides have potentially harmful side-effects. Some have more, some have less, and some may have long-term side-effects which are yet to be determined. But all experts now agree that drugs should be used to lower cholesterol only after a determined – but failed – effort has been made to lower LDL cholesterol enough to move out of the high-risk-for-heart-disease category.

Also, drugs work better in combination with a low-fat diet, and doctors want people to take the lowest dose possible of any drug they prescribe. Experts say that, for most people, a low-fat diet and treatment with a single drug – usually either a resin or a statin (we explain both below) – work well.

Q   **How high does cholesterol need to be for a doctor to prescribe drugs?**
A   Here are some guidelines:

• For people who already have heart disease, an LDL cholesterol level of more than 130 mg/dL. The goal is to reduce LDL to 100 mg/dL or lower.
• For people without heart disease but two or more other risk factors, an LDL level greater than 160 mg/dL. The goal is to reduce LDL to 130 mg/dL or lower.
• For people without heart disease and fewer than two other risk factors, an LDL cholesterol level of 190 mg/dL. The goal is to reduce LDL to 160 mg/dL or lower.

Q   **And what about triglycerides?**
A   High triglycerides are almost always found along with high LDL cholesterol. In that case, triglycerides need to

be 200 mg/dL or higher for your doctor to consider using drugs.

If you have high triglycerides alone – a genetic condition – drug treatment is usually started at 500 mg/dL or so, depending on your other risk factors.

Q   **These recommendations sound very positive. Are they engraved in stone?**

A   Definitely not. In reality, the cut-off point at which drugs are clearly required is different for each person, so the decision whether to start drugs may be a complicated one. Doctors need to take the severity of other risk factors into consideration. Someone with severe diabetes or high blood pressure, for instance, is a more likely candidate for immediate drug therapy than someone who is slightly overweight and sedentary. And your age and whether you're a man or woman are always relevant factors. That's where your doctor's individual management and advice come in.

Q   **So not everyone needs to take drugs even though their LDL cholesterol levels remain a bit high?**

A   Correct. If you're not considered to be at high risk of developing heart disease over the next one or two decades, drug therapy will often be withheld or delayed – even if your LDL cholesterol or triglycerides are higher than they should be. That may be the case for pre-menopausal women, and men under the age of 35.

On the other hand, if you are considered to be at very high risk – if your LDL cholesterol level is well over

220 mg/dL, you have multiple risk factors or established heart disease – your doctor may want to start you on cholesterol- or triglyceride-lowering drugs shortly after starting dietary therapy. He or she is most likely to do this if it is believed you won't be able to reduce your levels enough through dietary changes alone.

Q **So my doctor's beliefs about cholesterol-lowering diet and drugs might have something to do with what he or she recommends to me?**

A It might have a lot to do with it.

More doctors than ever are prescribing cholesterol-lowering drugs, especially the newer, stronger drugs known as the statins because of the findings of a study described in Chapter 2, the so-called '4-S' study – the Scandinavian Simvastatin Survival Study.

In this study, a drug, simvastatin (Zocor), performed impressively. It reduced the overall risk of death by 30 per cent and decreased the risk of death from heart attack by 42 per cent. It also cut people's risk of having to undergo bypass surgery, and it reduced risks in women of any age and in people over the age of 60, two groups for which the benefits of cholesterol-lowering drug therapy have been less than certain. Because of these impressive findings, Zocor's maker, Merck & Co., have been authorized to re-label this drug the first anti-cholesterol drug which actually reduces deaths from heart disease. And some doctors are urging heart patients to get their cholesterol levels re-checked and to consider trying this drug if their LDL cholesterol hasn't dropped to 100 mg/dL with other treatments.

But some doctors believe the potential risks of even these new, apparently safer cholesterol-lowering drugs have been underplayed, and that long-term risks may yet emerge. These doctors are more reserved in prescribing. They believe cholesterol-lowering drugs should be used only for people with established heart disease whose cholesterol cannot be controlled by diet alone. And these doctors may be very aggressive about lowering your cholesterol and triglycerides with diet, and with lowering your other risks for heart disease with lifestyle changes, such as stopping smoking, losing weight and exercising.

An editorial in the *British Medical Journal* of 20 May, 1995 states that, following the Scandinavian simvastatin survival study, 'There is no longer any doubt about the benefit and safety of treating hypercholesterolaemia in patients who have had a myocardial infarction [heart attack].' So far as primary prevention is concerned, however, the writers believed that conservatism was still justified.

Q   **Tell me again, how long am I supposed to be trying this diet and lifestyle stuff?**

A   At least three months, and doctors who are the most successful at getting results with diet say up to a year, or even longer if you are continuing to improve. As mentioned in Chapter 5, it takes time to incorporate healthier habits into your life. If your cholesterol is high and you are serious about avoiding drugs and heart disease, you have little choice but to go along with a diet and lifestyle programme.

Q **What if I am already taking cholesterol-lowering drugs?**
A They aren't necessarily a lifetime sentence. You may be able to reduce the dose or get off the drugs altogether (with medical supervision) if you can reduce your risks, including high cholesterol, with a renewed attempt at lifestyle changes.

Q **What kinds of drugs are used to treat cholesterol?**
A Bile acid binding resins (see below) eliminate cholesterol from the body. These drugs were also mentioned in Chapter 4, since they are the only cholesterol-lowering drugs approved for use in children. There are also drugs which block the liver's production of cholesterol. These include two major classes of drugs, the statin drugs and the fibric acid derivatives (see page 116 and 119). Also capable of blocking the production of cholesterol is a form of the B vitamin niacin (called nicotinic acid) (see page 110).

BILE ACID BINDING RESINS

Q **What are bile acid binding resins?**
A Well, for one thing, they are man-made resins. They are gritty, insoluble granules which come as a powder to be mixed with a liquid, or as a bar that has to be chewed thoroughly. These resins bind with the cholesterol-rich

bile acids secreted by the liver, preventing cholesterol from being reabsorbed into your body. Instead, it passes out of your body in the faeces. These drugs are also often called bile acid sequestrants, since they sequester, or isolate, bile acid.

Q   **How does that lower cholesterol in the blood?**
A   Every day, a considerable quantity of cholesterol comes down the bile duct into the intestine. Normally, most of this cholesterol is reabsorbed into the bloodstream and is circulated back to the liver. Binding resins capture this bile cholesterol and convert it to a form which cannot be reabsorbed into the blood. When this normal recycling of bile acid back to the liver is inhibited, stores of cholesterol in the cells in the liver necessarily drop. The cells respond by drawing in more cholesterol from the blood to make bile acid. This results in a drop in both total and LDL cholesterol and a small increase in protective HDL cholesterol.

Q   **How much of a drop can I expect to see using a bile acid binding resin?**
A   Both of the bile acid binding resins available, cholestyramine (Questran, a powder) and colestipol (Cholybar, a chewable bar and Colestid, granules) are equally effective in lowering LDL cholesterol.

People taking a normal daily dose can expect their LDL cholesterol to drop by 15 to 25 per cent, depending on how high it is before they start taking the drug.

Q   **What kinds of people take these drugs?**

A   As detailed below, these drugs have a long safety record and seldom cause serious side-effects. So they are a first choice for most people with high LDL cholesterol – men, women and sometimes children with cholesterol-elevating genetic disorders.

Some doctors also recommend bile acid resins for young adults, particularly men, with high LDL cholesterol levels but no other risk factors for heart disease, because of their increased odds of dying from heart disease later in life.

Q   **Are these drugs actually proven to reduce someone's chances of developing heart disease?**

A   Yes. In the Lipid Research Clinic's Coronary Primary Prevention trial of the mid-1980s they were shown to reduce the risk of coronary heart disease.

Q   **What kinds of side-effects do bile acid binding resins have?**

A   These drugs are not absorbed into the body, so they have fewer side-effects than other cholesterol-lowering drugs.

However, they can adversely affect the bowels. This drug makes the stools dense and sticky, so two out of three people develop constipation, and some develop severe constipation and even faecal impaction – hardened or putty-like stools stuck in the rectum or colon.

How constipated someone gets depends on the dose. If he or she is taking only two scoops, packets or bars a day, constipation is less than if taking four or six doses. Constipation is also more likely, and more severe, in older people.

Q   What can one do for the constipation? Take laxatives?
A   Laxative pills are better avoided, since regular use can deplete the body of nutrients. But there are safe and effective osmotic agents which retain water in the intestine so as to soften the stools. If these are taken along with plenty of water they will alleviate most of the symptoms of constipation caused by bile acid binding resins.

    Other complaints associated with this class of drugs include abdominal pain, heartburn, nausea, belching and bloating.

Q   Any other side-effects?
A   The bile acid sequestering drugs can also interfere with the absorption of other medications you take, so other drugs should be taken at least one hour before the bile acid binding resin, or, if this is not possible, four hours afterwards.

    The drugs also interfere with the absorption of the fat-soluble vitamins – A, D, E and K – and folic acid and iron. So if you're taking vitamin supplements, take them with a meal when you are not taking a bile acid sequestering drug, or four hours after your last dose.

Q   Can these drugs cause vitamin deficiencies?
A   At the usual dosages they are not known to cause vitamin- or mineral-deficiency related problems, such as

anaemia. Vitamin deficiencies can be hard to detect, however – especially for fat-soluble vitamins – and doctors often don't even think to look for them. So keep a lookout yourself. Signs of deficiency of these nutrients may include depression, easy bruising or bleeding (including nosebleeds), fatigue, weakened immunity, dry eyes, night blindness and bone pain.

Q   **Any other side-effects I should know about?**
A   Sometimes blood triglycerides rise when you take a bile acid binding resin. The increase may be transient, but it persists in some people and may require the use of a second lipid-lowering drug, such as nicotinic acid, which we describe next, to lower triglyceride levels.

NIACIN (NICOTINIC ACID)

Q   **I've heard that a vitamin, niacin, is used to lower cholesterol. What can you tell me about it?**
A   Only one form of niacin, nicotinic acid, can lower cholesterol. Another form, nicotinamide, has no effect on cholesterol.

Q   **Nicotinic acid. Isn't that found in cigarettes?**
A   No. Despite similarities in names, nicotinic acid is not related to nicotine, the addictive substance found in tobacco.

Q   **How do I get nicotinic acid? In foods?**
A   While there's some in foods, there's nowhere near

enough to lower your cholesterol. Most people get only 15 to 35 mg of niacin a day from foods. At least 60 times that amount is required (as nicotinic acid) to help lower cholesterol. The usual dosage is 0.5 to 0.75 grams a day, with a recommended maximum of 1.2 grams daily, although as much as 6 grams a day has been prescribed. You can get nicotinic acid without a prescription, but never take large doses without medical supervision. A nicotinic acid derivative prescribed in Britain is acipimox (Olbetam).

Q   How does it work?
A   Its main action is in the liver, where it interferes with the manufacture of cholesterol, probably in several ways, through mechanisms which are not well understood. Its effect on the liver leads to decreased production of triglyceride-rich VLDL cholesterol. And since VLDL cholesterol is eventually converted to LDL cholesterol, nicotinic acid reduces both LDL cholesterol and triglyceride levels.

Q   How much of a reduction can I expect to see?
A   The higher your cholesterol to begin with, the more of a drop you'll see. People with total cholesterol of 240 mg/dL or higher might see a 10 to 20 per cent drop in total cholesterol and in LDL cholesterol levels, a reduction comparable to that achieved with normal doses of 20 to 40 mg a day of lovastatin, a drug we talk about in a minute.
    Nicotinic acid also reduces blood levels of two proteins thought to be linked with heart disease:

homocysteine and methylmalonic acid, which are also reduced by folic acid.

Q   **What about HDL cholesterol? Does nicotinic acid affect it?**

A   Yes. Nicotinic acid has the greatest HDL-raising effect of any drug. In gram doses, it increases HDL cholesterol levels by an average of 20 to 35 per cent.

That's good, because studies suggest that a 1 mg/dL increase in HDL cholesterol levels should decrease the risk of coronary heart disease by 2 to 3 per cent. By reducing LDL and increasing HDL cholesterol levels, nicotinic acid can improve people's HDL-to-total-cholesterol ratio, a figure which some doctors think is the best indicator of your risk of developing heart disease.

Q   **So should I take nicotinic acid if my total cholesterol is normal but my HDLs are low?**

A   Experts are inclined to advise against drug therapy for people with normal total or LDL cholesterol levels but low HDLs. Exercise can raise HDLs. We talk more about exercise in Chapter 7.

Q   **Has nicotinic acid been proved to reduce the risk of heart disease?**

A   Yes. It has a fairly impressive history. One study, the Coronary Drug Project, suggested that nicotinic acid can protect against heart disease both while it's being used and long after it's stopped, something no other drug has been shown to do. In a follow-up 10 years after the initial five-year study ended, those who had taken 2 grams a day of nicotinic acid had 20 per cent less coronary heart disease than a corresponding group who had taken a placebo.

Q **Now give me the bad news. What are the side-effects?**
A Nicotinic acid has been around for a while. It was first found to lower cholesterol back in 1955, and it has been used extensively for at least 20 years, so most of its side-effects are known.

    The most common side-effect is something called the niacin flush. About half an hour after you take it, you'll feel warmth, flushing and itchiness, usually on your face and upper body. This effect lasts only 15 to 30 minutes.

Q **Any way to get round this?**
A Doctors say that, in most people, the flush is worst when they first start taking the drug – one good reason to start it on a weekend – and that it soon lessens as the body adapts to the drug.

    And the flush can be greatly minimized if you gradually increase your dose of nicotinic acid, starting with as little as 100 mg, three times a day, slowly increasing the dose until you reach your initial target level, usually 250 mg, three times a day. Taking nicotinic acid with a meal also helps. So does taking one ordinary aspirin tablet with the nicotinic acid. Avoid taking the drug with alcohol or hot drinks, which usually make the flush worse.

Q Aren't there more serious side-effects associated with nicotinic acid? I heard it can cause liver problems.

A It can. A regular dose can cause problems, but the time-release form, which causes less flushing, is even more likely to cause this potentially serious side-effect. Only the time-release form, however, in amounts of 500 mg or more a day, has been reported to cause severe, permanent liver damage. Most doctors don't recommend time-release nicotinic acid for this reason.

Q How can nicotinic acid cause liver damage?

A In the large doses used to lower cholesterol, nicotinic acid can irritate liver cells. If it's going to do this, it usually does soon after you start the drug. A doctor can check for liver damage by testing your blood for certain enzymes released by the liver – a liver function test. This test should be done four to six weeks after you have reached your initial target dose, usually about 0.75 to 1 gram daily of the nicotinic acid derivative acipimox, and then on a regular basis.

Q What's a typical dose?

A Acipimox (Olbetam) is given in 250 mg (0.25 gram) capsules in a dose of, usually, two or three capsules a day. It is not given to children.

Q Does nicotinic acid ever cause permanent liver damage?

A Usually not. The changes in liver function usually last only a few weeks and are moderate in degree. But sometimes people do have a severe reaction to nicotinic acid and have to stop taking it. Even then, their livers usually recover in two to three months. Occasionally people start taking nicotinic acid again and have no problems with it. Still, they need to be monitored carefully.

Note, however, that in Britain it is the nicotinic acid derivative acipimox which is normally prescribed. Liver problems are not reported with this form.

Q   So I guess people with liver problems shouldn't take nicotinic acid?

A   It's generally not prescribed for people with severe or unexplained liver problems, and should be used only with caution in people with a history of stomach or intestinal ulcers. If you have an active ulcer, you shouldn't be taking it at all. The same applies even for the nicotinic acid derivative acipimox.

If you tend to have gout attacks, nicotinic acid may not be the best cholesterol-lowering drug for you, since it can increase blood levels of uric acid and bring on an attack of gout. During an attack, blood levels of uric acid get so high that some of it crystallizes in joints, causing acute pain.

And people with diabetes must be carefully monitored if they take this drug, since it can make their blood-sugar levels harder to control.

Q   Do you need a prescription to take nicotinic acid?

A   No. Nicotinic acid can be obtained without prescription at a chemist's or health-food shop. But because of the possible side-effects, it's important that you do not take large amounts of nicotinic acid without medical supervision. If you really need a drug in this category, you will be better off with a prescription for acipimox.

STATIN DRUGS

Q   I've heard there are some strong new drugs which can really lower cholesterol. What are they?

A   You're referring to a class of drugs called the statins because their chemical names all end in 'statin'. These drugs are officially called **HMG CoA reductase inhibitors**, and they include lovastatin (Mevacor), the oldest of these drugs, marketed since 1982, and other closely related newcomers such as atorvastatin (Lipitor), pravastatin (Lipostat), simvastatin (Zocor) and fluvastatin (Lescol).

Q   How do these drugs work?

A   Like nicotinic acid, drugs in this class work in the liver to block the manufacture of cholesterol. They do this by inhibiting the action of a key enzyme involved in cholesterol production, called HMG CoA reductase. As the amount of cholesterol being produced in the liver drops, the cells in the liver take up more LDL cholesterol from the blood, so blood levels of LDL cholesterol drop.

Q   How much of a drop in cholesterol levels can I expect to see with these drugs?

A   That depends on your dosage and how high your

cholesterol was to begin with. Generally, though, studies show a 20 to 30 per cent drop in both total and LDL cholesterol levels. Triglycerides also drop with these drugs, from 7 to 20 per cent. And HDL cholesterol increases, from 6 to 12 per cent.

Q How does this compare with the other drugs already discussed?

A All indications are that the statin drugs work at least as well as the bile acid binding resins and nicotinic acid in preventing coronary heart disease.

It was a statin drug (simvastatin, used in the '4-S' study) which caused a reduced risk of 30 per cent from death from any cause, and a reduced risk of 42 per cent from death caused by a heart attack.

Q Is simvastatin better than the other statin drugs?

A No tests have been done to detect differences in the ability to lower cholesterol among these drugs, presumably because the pharmaceutical companies believe they are quite similar. But most of the work that has been done on these drugs indicates that they work equally well at lowering cholesterol.

On a milligram-per-milligram basis, simvastatin appears to be most potent, but equivalent cholesterol reductions can be achieved with the other agents if higher doses are used.

Q **What about side-effects? Are they the same in all these drugs?**
A They seem to be, although since lovastatin has been around the longest, more is known about its long-term side-effects than for the other drugs.

Q **What are the side-effects?**
A They are numerous, they can be serious and some doctors believe not all the long-term side-effects of these drugs have been revealed as yet.

Out of every 100 people who take these drugs, about 2 will have liver function problems. So everyone taking these drugs needs to undergo liver function tests about four to six weeks after they start taking the drugs, and then twice a year.

Muscle inflammation with partial destruction of muscle cells – a condition known as rhabdomyolysis – is also a serious side-effect, reported in about 1 in 100 people taking these drugs. Its incidence increases when statin drugs are combined with other drugs, including gemfibrozil, nicotinic acid, cyclosporin and erythromycin. So you'll need to avoid these drugs if possible.

Since this problem can be associated with the breakdown of muscle tissue and, along with it, kidney failure, it is vitally important to tell your doctor if you develop weak or tender muscles, backache or what seems like 'rheumatism' or excess muscle stiffness after exercise.

Blood tests that measure the by-products of muscle breakdown should be done regularly to alert your doctor to early signs of inflammation.

Q   Any other side-effects?

A   Constipation, diarrhoea, flatulence and nausea can occur, although these symptoms are less common than with the bile acid binding resins. Headaches, dizziness and blurred vision are also possible.

In animals – taking much higher doses of the drugs than would normally be given – lovastatin has produced optic-nerve degeneration and lesions in the central nervous system. However, these nerve problems have not been noted in people taking the drug.

Q   Is it possible I shouldn't take one of these drugs?

A   Of course. Since there are so many potential side-effects, you should think twice about using any of them. You may be able to reduce your cholesterol sufficiently using diet, bile acid binding resins, and perhaps some nicotinic acid or acipimox. If your cholesterol is in the 200 to 240 mg/dL range, you should weigh up the risks of taking these drugs against their potential benefits.

The manufacturers say these drugs should be 'prescribed with caution' to people with liver disease or possible liver or kidney problems, women who are breast-feeding, pregnant women, and women of childbearing age unless they are highly unlikely to become pregnant.

FIBRIC ACID DERIVATIVES

Q   What are fibric acid derivatives?

A   Also known as fibrates, these are cholesterol- and triglyc-eride-lowering drugs that have been around since the late 1960s. They were initially prescribed with some enthusiasm because they seemed to have fewer side-effects than bile acid resins and nicotinic acid – the two other serious contenders at the time – but they were found to have their own very serious side-effects. So today they are prescribed only for certain conditions, which will be described on page 122 .

Q   What are the names of these drugs?

A   Several fibric acid derivatives are currently available in Britain: gemfibrozil (Lopid), clofibrate (Atromid-S), bezafibrate (Bezalid Mono), fenofibrate (Lipantil Micro) and ciprofibrate (Modalim).

Q   How do fibric acid derivatives lower cholesterol?

A   They work in the liver, but the way they work is not well understood. They increase the liver's ability to break down VLDL cholesterol, which drops triglyceride levels. And they raise HDL cholesterol levels slightly.

Q   So what is the problem with these drugs?

A   It's true that these drugs have been shown to reduce the risk of fatal and non-fatal heart attacks in two large studies of people with no signs of heart disease. However, there was an increase in total deaths in people taking clofibrate in one of these studies, the World Health Organization trial. In the other study, the Helsinki Heart Study, gemfibrozil did not cause an increase in deaths during the study, but in an $8^1/_2$-year follow-up the people who had taken gemfibrozil during the study had a 20 per cent increased rate of death compared with the placebo group.

As a result of these findings, prescriptions of clofibrate and its closely related cousin, gemfibrozil, have dropped off considerably.

Q   **What happens to people who take these drugs?**
A   With clofibrate, half the deaths were due to malignancies, such as liver cancer. Some were due to gallbladder disease or complications from gallbladder surgery. Other studies have reported an increase in heart arrhythmia, blood clotting and angina in people taking clofibrate.

Q   **And with gemfibrozil?**
A   Because it's so closely related to clofibrate, it is considered to have the same potential risk for toxicity, including cancer and gallbladder problems, plus an increased risk of death not linked to heart disease.

Q   **What about less serious side-effects?**
A   The list is long: stomach upset, nausea, diarrhoea, rash, muscle pain, weakness, liver function problems, dizziness and blurred vision are just some of the potential side-effects.

Q   **So whom are these drugs prescribed for these days – masochists?**
A   Clofibrate or gemfibrozil may be prescribed for people who have very high triglyceride levels – 2,000 mg/dL or more – as the result of genetic disorders. These people

may also be at high risk of developing pancreatitis, a serious, painful inflammation of the pancreas.

Gemfibrozil is prescribed more often than clofibrate, and may also be used to prevent the development of heart disease in people with a combination of high LDL cholesterol, high triglycerides and low HDL cholesterol. However, benefits from the drug seem to be limited to people with LDL/HDL ratios of more than 5:1 and triglycerides higher than 200 mg/dL.

Q By how much do these drugs reduce triglycerides?

A They reduce triglycerides by 20 to 50 per cent while increasing HDL cholesterol 10 to 15 per cent. But they don't lower LDL cholesterol very much – only 10 to 15 per cent.

Q Do doctors ever prescribe combinations of cholesterol drugs? Is this more dangerous than using only one?

A Drugs are sometimes combined to treat very high cholesterol or in an attempt to keep dosages low. Some combinations give good results.

For instance, either nicotinic acid or statin drugs can be used along with bile acid binding resins without added side-effects. In the case of statin drugs, this may allow someone to take the smallest dosage of this drug, 20 mg a day. Used alone, this would result in an average drop in LDL cholesterol of 24 per cent. But used in combination with the lowest dose of a bile acid binding resin, LDL cholesterol drops by up to 43 per cent. Of course, a patient needs to take each of these drugs separately during the day, since the bile acid binding resin can interfere with the body's ability to absorb the statin drug.

Some combinations can be dangerous, however, and are not used. Combining nicotinic acid and a statin drug, or two statin drugs, for instance, may lead to an increased risk of serious muscle inflammation.

Q **How do I know if my doctor is prescribing the right drug, or drugs, for me?**

A Ask your doctor why he or she is prescribing a particular drug for you. Is it because your triglycerides are particularly high? Because your HDLs are low? Because your LDLs are still much too high after a year or more of changing your lifestyle and diet?

Ask what the drug is expected to do and how you will be monitored for side-effects. Make sure your doctor knows of any other drugs you are taking, prescription or non-prescription. Ask about any possible interactions. You want to make sure your doctor is making a decision based on your individual needs, not on the last drug company salesperson who was in the consulting room.

When you go to have your prescription made up, ask the chemist for an information sheet on your drug. Make sure you get the real thing, not an abbreviated patient information sheet. Read it and keep it on hand to refer to later, if necessary, for possible side-effects.

This information is also available in books such as the latest editions of the *British National Formulary* or *Martindale's the Extra Pharmacopoeia*. Most libraries have copies of these books in their reference section.

CHAPTER SEVEN

OTHER FACTORS THAT AFFECT CHOLESTEROL AND HEART DISEASE

Q   You mentioned some other risk factors for heart disease – smoking, stress, lack of exercise and the like. Why are these risk factors? Do they raise cholesterol levels?

A   All of them can contribute to heart disease in a number of ways: by causing the oxidation of LDL cholesterol, making blood quicker to clot, damaging artery linings, causing blood vessel constriction and raising cholesterol levels or lowering HDL cholesterol.

SMOKING

Q   I know smoking is bad for the heart. But how bad? And why?

A   Cigarette smoking is an important risk factor for heart disease for everyone – men and women – of any age. Heart attacks are $2^1/_2$ times more common in smokers than in non-smokers. A comparable increase in risk would come from having a cholesterol level of 300 mg/dL or more. Smoking also takes away a woman's pre-menopausal protection from oestrogen, the main female hormone, since it depletes oestrogen in the body.

Q But what if I don't smoke all that much?

A It's true that the risk increases with the number of cigarettes you smoke each day. But if you smoke even 20 a day, your risk of heart disease is twice as high as that of someone who has never smoked. That risk is comparable to a total cholesterol level of 300 mg/dL.

If you smoke 40 or more cigarettes a day, your risk is three times as high as that of a person who has never smoked. Cigars, pipes and chewing tobacco also increase your risk – by perhaps as much as two times that of a person who has never smoked. And the earlier in life you start smoking, the more negative an impact it is likely to have on your health.

Q Does smoking low-tar and low-nicotine cigarettes reduce my risk of heart disease?

A Sorry, no. While these cigarettes may reduce your risk of cancer, they have not been proved to reduce your risk of heart disease. Studies show that people who smoke low-tar and low-nicotine cigarettes often inhale more deeply, hold their breath after inhaling, and smoke more cigarettes in an unconscious effort to maintain the nicotine levels to which their bodies are addicted. Consequently, they do not reduce their nicotine exposure as much as they may have hoped and also inhale more of the other toxic substances contained in the smoke.

Q **How exactly does smoking affect the heart?**

A Smoking causes the oxidation of lipids, the first step in the process of plaque build-up. It reduces the ratio of HDL to LDL cholesterol and increases the tendency for blood to clot inside the blood vessels and obstruct blood flow. Constituents of tobacco smoke also directly damage endothelial cells, the cells lining the inside of blood vessels.

Q **Sounds bad.**

A It is. And cigarette smoking also has temporary adverse effects on the heart and blood vessels, and these may provoke serious consequences, such as heart attacks. The nicotine in smoke increases blood pressure and heart rate. Carbon monoxide, a gas produced by smoking – the same gas in car exhaust which is lethal in an enclosed space – gets into the blood and reduces the amount of oxygen blood can carry to the heart and the rest of the body. It causes arteries in the arms and legs to constrict, and can cause a lack of oxygen and blood flow to the heart muscle by temporarily decreasing the diameter of the coronary arteries.

Q **If someone gives up smoking, how long will it take for the risk of heart disease to drop?**

A Not long. A major reduction in risk occurs within the first year after stopping, and the risk drops dramatically within about two years. Although the risk never drops to where it would be if you had never smoked, it will eventually drop so that it's only about one-third higher.

Q   **What if I've been smoking for years? Does it really help to stop?**

A   Yes! For example, if you are older than 50 and stop smoking, your chance of dying from any cause is reduced by one-half during the next 15 years. And your risk of dying of heart disease decreases by about 30 per cent.

Q   **I don't smoke, but I'm exposed to cigarette smoke all day long at work. Does that increase my risk of heart disease?**

A   Yes. Studies find that exposure to cigarette smoke in the workplace or at home increases your risk of heart disease by a factor of 20 to 70 per cent. In fact, passive smoking has a stronger link with heart disease than it does with lung cancer.

EXERCISE

Q   **I've heard exercise is supposed to help prevent heart disease? Does it?**

A   Yes. Sedentary people have nearly twice the risk of having a fatal heart attack as active people when other factors are equal.

Q   **What does it mean to be sedentary?**

A   You are sedentary if you have a job that is inactive or spend most of your day sitting and do not take time to exercise for 20 to 30 minutes at least three times a week.

Q   **Is 20 to 30 minutes three times a week all that's required to protect your heart?**

A   Not necessarily. It's simply enough to move you out of the 'couch potato' category. Studies suggest that the best protection comes from getting four or five hours a week of aerobic exercise – the huff-and-puff kind.

Q   **How does exercise protect your heart? Does it lower cholesterol?**

A   Regular exercise raises blood levels of 'good' HDL cholesterol. How much it goes up by depends on your initial cholesterol level, age, weight and amount of body fat, as well as the intensity of your workouts.

Q   **How much of an increase can someone expect to see?**

A   Endurance athletes, such as long-distance runners or swimmers, often have HDL levels which are 10 to 24 mg/dL higher than those of people who don't exercise at all. And studies also indicate that moderate exercise, such as walking briskly for an hour three times a week, also raises HDLs.

Q   **Does exercise do anything else to help prevent heart disease?**

A   If it helps you lose weight, you'll also probably have a drop in LDL cholesterol and triglycerides and you may reduce your risk of developing diabetes or high blood pressure, two other big risk factors for heart disease.

Aerobic exercise strengthens your heart muscle, making it pump more blood with each beat. Exercise also makes the platelets in your blood less sticky, which helps to reduce the possibility of blood clotting in the arteries. And in animals, at least, regular exercise stimulates the formation of collateral coronary arteries, providing blood supply to the heart by going around blockages. Whether this also happens in humans is not known for sure, but there are indications that it does.

Q It sounds as if everyone should exercise. But don't people who already have heart disease drop dead when they start running?

A It's true that exercise can precipitate sudden cardiac death, especially in people with known heart disease.

But according to two studies such cases are rare, even though they often make the headlines. Most at risk are so-called 'weekend warriors', people who throw themselves into strenuous activity without first taking the time to get into shape. People who exercise regularly also increase their risk of dying during peak exertion, but their overall risk of sudden death is actually 60 per cent lower than for people who never exercise. So the exercise really *is* protecting their hearts.

STRESS

Q Is it true that a person can get so stressed out that he or she has a heart attack?

A Yes. It's not uncommon for people with heart disease to report that emotional peaks cause chest pain. And it's common for heart attacks to occur during emotionally difficult times. However, most people who have stress-related heart symptoms have underlying atherosclerosis.

Q   **Can stress cause the development of heart disease?**
A   That's not entirely clear, in part because stress – and people's reactions to it – are so hard to study and measure. Some doctors believe that stress plays a major role in the development of heart disease and heart attacks.

    One recent study, for instance, found that men who rated themselves as highly anxious back in 1961 were three to four times more likely to go on to have a sudden fatal heart attack than men who rated themselves as low in anxiety.

Q   **Does stress raise cholesterol levels?**
A   Some doctors claim no. But a recent study found just the opposite. The researchers determined that within 20 minutes of starting on a frustrating mental task, people had an increase of up to 5 mg/dL in total cholesterol, with a slightly lower rise in triglycerides, HDL and LDL cholesterol.

Q   **Can't stress also hurt my heart in other ways?**
A   Apparently so. The biochemicals your body released during stress trigger processes which can harm the artery walls. They can also make blood thicker and more prone to clotting.

    Stress raises blood pressure and blood-sugar levels, speeds up the heart rate, contributes to heartbeat irregularities (arrhythmia) and causes blood vessels to constrict. It can even produce coronary spasms, thus narrowing the arteries and reducing the flow of blood to the heart. Mental stress, especially anger, has been reported to trigger angina, heart attacks and even sudden death.

Q **What can I do if I'm under stress or tend to overreact to things?**

A For a start, take good care of yourself. Don't smoke or stuff yourself on fatty foods. Exercise is a great way to reduce stress. It actually uses up the 'fight or flight' biochemicals produced in a stressful episode – adrenaline-like chemicals.

Yoga, meditation, spiritual pursuits, learned relaxation techniques, talking it out with a friend or therapist, social activities and just plain having fun are good ways to diffuse stress.

OVERWEIGHT

Q **Does being overweight raise cholesterol levels?**

A It can. People who are obese (more than 20 per cent overweight) do tend to have higher LDL and lower HDL cholesterol than people who are not overweight. But excess body fat doesn't necessarily cause these cholesterol changes. It may simply be found along with them. People who are obese also tend to have other risk factors for heart disease: high triglyceride levels, high blood sugar, high blood pressure, diabetes.

Q   So does being obese increase my chances of having a heart attack?

A   Study findings are mixed on this. Because obesity is so often found along with the other risk factors just mentioned, it's hard to know if obesity, in itself, is a risk for heart disease. Some research seems to suggest that if your only risk is being fat – no high blood pressure or cholesterol, no diabetes – you're probably not at increased risk. Other studies find that even a slight increase in weight – 10 to 15 pounds – raises your risk. Take your pick.

Q   I've heard that having a pot belly increases risk of heart disease more than being fat all over. Is that true?

A   Yes. Many women have fat on their hips and thighs, which is not associated with increased risk, whereas pot bellies (visceral fat) on men or women are linked with heart disease. People with pot bellies often also have high insulin and high blood-sugar levels, which also contribute to heart disease.

Q   Does losing weight help to reduce my risk of heart disease?

A   It does if you have other risk factors associated with obesity. If you can lose weight and keep it off you may be able to eliminate all the risk factors just mentioned. Losing weight is often the only thing that's needed to reverse late-onset diabetes and high triglycerides. And losing just 5 or 10 pounds can double the reduction you'll see in LDL cholesterol on a low-saturated-fat diet.

Q **Do thin people ever have high cholesterol or atherosclerosis?**

A Yes. While overweight people are about twice as likely as thin people to have high cholesterol, thin people can also have high cholesterol. Usually this is the result of an inherited abnormality in cholesterol metabolism, which can make their high cholesterol more difficult than normal to treat.

RACE

Q **What about race? Are white people more vulnerable to heart disease than black people?**

A No, the opposite is true. Heart disease death rates are up to 70 per cent higher among blacks than among whites of the same age, at least up until the age of 74, when it evens out. The reason for this difference is not entirely clear, but it apparently does not have to do with higher cholesterol levels, since HDL cholesterol is actually higher in blacks than in whites.

It may be that black people are more likely than white people to have other additional risk factors. They continue to smoke more than whites, for instance, and a higher percentage have high blood pressure or diabetes.

Q   **Heart disease – even just one aspect of it, cholesterol – is more complicated than I ever thought. How am I supposed to remember all this stuff, much less do anything about it?**

A   Don't despair. Just keep in mind these points:

- Know your figures. But remember, high cholesterol is not heart disease; it is not even a guarantee that you'll get heart disease. It is simply a measure of risk. Make sure your cholesterol is measured accurately; ask your doctor to tell you specifically how your figures affect your risk of heart disease. Ask for copies of your tests and of your medical records, which should also include other figures you need to know – blood pressure, blood sugar and your weight.

- Know your other risk factors for heart disease and be prepared to change the top two or three. Persist in getting the help you need. Ask your doctor about help in stopping smoking, beginning exercise, or dieting. If necessary, he or she can prescribe nicotine gum or patches and refer you to specialists for additional help. Such professionals may also be able to help you devise tactics for stress reduction and weight control.

- Even a one-time referral to a physiotherapist can help you to get started on an exercise programme. Or, if you already have heart disease, ask about enrolling in a cardiac-rehabilitation programme. Find out what your local hospital has to offer in the way of heart disease prevention programmes (known as

'wellness' programmes, in some cases). At your
favourite health-food shop get advice about local
alternative healthcare professionals. But check them
out at least as carefully as you would any healthcare
provider.

- Improve your diet if necessary. There are many
books available on the subject.
- Stay as up to date as you can by continuing to read
about heart disease and cholesterol. If you read
about a particularly interesting study in the newspa-
per, go to the nearest hospital library and read the
original study, usually published in a professional
journal. And ask your doctor what he or she thinks
about it the next time you visit the surgery.

GLOSSARY

ABSOLUTE RISK
Actual risk; your 'odds', as in 1 in 100.

ANGINA PECTORIS
Chest pain, often with an accompanying feeling of suffocation, caused by insufficient oxygen to the heart muscle.

ANTIOXIDANT
A substance with the ability to interfere with oxygen-generated, or oxidative, reactions caused by free radicals. **Low-density lipoprotein** (LDL) cholesterol, for instance, undergoes **oxidation** as part of the early stages of **atherosclerosis**.

APOLIPOPROTEINS
Any of the protein constituents of lipoproteins; some apolipoproteins may prove to be markers for inherited cholesterol disorders.

ARTERIOGRAPHY

A test that can measure obstruction inside an artery.

ARTERIOSCLEROSIS

A broad, if somewhat old-fashioned, term used to cover a variety of diseases, including **atherosclerosis**, which lead to abnormal thickening and hardening of the walls of the arteries.

ATHEROSCLEROSIS

The principal arterial disease and the largest single cause of premature death and disability in the developed world. It features a gradual build-up of fatty deposits, called **plaques**, on the inside walls of the arteries. These limit blood flow to those organs which the arteries supply. Total obstruction may occur as blood clots on top of a plaque. This is how heart attacks and strokes occur.

ATTRIBUTABLE RISK

The amount of risk that can be pinned on a specific risk factor, such as smoking.

BETA-CAROTENE

An orange pigment, found in vegetables and fruits, which acts as an antioxidant in the body and which helps to regenerate vitamin E.

BILE ACID BINDING RESINS
Cholesterol-lowering drugs which act by binding with cholesterol-laden bile in the intestines, making it unabsorbable.

CALCIFICATION
The gathering of calcium deposits in body tissue. These deposits harden arteries.

CANOLA OIL
A bland, light-coloured vegetable oil from rapeseed which is mostly monounsaturated fats. These fats drop LDL cholesterol levels.

CAROTID ULTRASOUND TEST
A noninvasive test which uses sound waves to measure the extent of calcium deposition and consequent hardening in the carotid arteries of the neck.

CEREBROVASCULAR DISEASE
Blockages or disruption of blood circulation in the brain, including stroke.

CHOLESTEROL
A white, waxy substance found naturally throughout the body, belonging to a class of compounds called **sterols**.

CHOLESTYRAMINE
A cholesterol-lowering drug; a **bile acid binding resin**.

CHYLOMICRONS
Tiny spheres of fat, mostly **triglycerides**, which go directly from the intestines to the liver and which are thought to have no direct effect on the development of atherosclerosis.

CLOFIBRATE (ATROMID-S)
A drug which lowers serum cholesterol by reducing **very low-density lipoprotein** (VLDL).

COLESTIPOL
A cholesterol-lowering drug; a **bile acid binding resin**.

COMPLETE LIPID PROFILE
A blood test that measures total cholesterol, **high-density lipoprotein** (HDL), triglycerides and, indirectly, LDL cholesterol.

CORONARY ARTERY DISEASE
Atherosclerosis and narrowing or blockage of the coronary arteries, the spaghetti-sized arteries which deliver blood to the muscle of the heart.

ELECTROCARDIOGRAPHY
A test that measures and records electrical activity in the heart.

ENDOTHELIAL CELLS
A layer of cells which lines and protects the inner surfaces of blood vessels.

FAMILIAL COMBINED HYPERLIPIDAEMIA (FCH)

An inherited disorder of both high cholesterol and triglycerides; a serious condition which affects about 1 per cent of the population and, if untreated, results in premature heart disease.

FAMILIAL HYPERCHOLESTEROLAEMIA (FH)

The most common form of inherited high cholesterol, caused by a defect in LDL receptors, the portals on cell membranes which allow cholesterol to move in and out.

FIBRIC ACID DERIVATIVES

A class of drugs that interfere with the body's ability to make cholesterol in the liver; includes **gemfibrozil** and **clofibrate**.

FOAM CELL

A large, foamy-looking type of immune cell – a **macrophage** – after it has eaten lots of cholesterol. Foam cells contribute to the development of atherosclerotic plaque.

GEMFIBROZIL (LOPID)

A lipid-regulating drug that decreases serum triglycerides and very low-density lipoprotein.

HIGH-DENSITY LIPOPROTEIN (HDL)

So-called 'good' cholesterol which helps to escort cholesterol from the body. High levels are linked with a reduced risk of heart disease.

HMG CoA REDUCTASE INHIBITORS

A class of drugs that interfere with the body's ability to make cholesterol in the liver; includes the statin drugs.

HYDROGENATED FATS

Oils processed so that hydrogen is added to their structure. This firms up the oil, but also makes it similar to saturated fats. Margarine and vegetable shortenings are hydrogenated fats.

LDL RECEPTORS

Portals on cell membranes which selectively allow LDL cholesterol to move in or out of a cell.

LINOLEIC ACID

One of two essential fatty acids which cannot be manufactured in the body, found only in vegetable oils such as canola, safflower and corn oil.

LINOLENIC ACID

One of two essential fatty acids which cannot be manufactured in the body, found only in vegetable oils such as canola, safflower and corn oil.

LIPID

A group of fats or fatty substances found in the body.

LIPOPROTEIN

A combination of lipids and protein.

LOW-DENSITY LIPOPROTEIN (LDL)
So-called 'bad' cholesterol. High levels of LDL cholesterol have been linked with an increased risk of heart disease.

MACROPHAGE
An immune cell which engulfs and consumes microorganisms and debris, including oxidized cholesterol.

MONOUNSATURATED FATS
Fats, such as olive or canola oil, which are only slightly saturated. Diets rich in monounsaturated fats have been linked with reduced levels of LDL cholesterol.

NIACIN
One of the B vitamins. One form of niacin, nicotinic acid, is used to lower cholesterol.

NICOTINIC ACID
A form of niacin, a B vitamin, used to lower cholesterol.

OCCLUSIVE PERIPHERAL VASCULAR DISEASE
Blockages of blood circulation in the legs or arms, causing intermittent claudication, a painful condition caused by obstruction to the flow of blood in arteries in the legs.

OMEGA-3 FATTY ACIDS
A form of fat, found in fatty fish and some plants, which may help to prevent heart disease.

OXIDATION

A chemical reaction that involves oxygen. LDL cholesterol becomes oxidized in the body in an early stage of atherosclerosis. Vitamin E and other antioxidant nutrients, such as vitamin C and beta-carotene, can limit oxidation.

PALMITIC ACID

The predominant saturated fat in red meat, butter fat, cottonseed and cocoa butter; it raises LDL cholesterol.

PANCREATITIS

Inflammation of the pancreas, often aggravated by super-high levels of triglycerides.

PLAQUE

A patch or flat area where cholesterol and other material has been deposited on an artery wall. Fatty plaques start the process of atherosclerosis.

PLATELET

A small, irregular structure, a fragment of a large cell, involved in blood coagulation.

PLATELET AGGREGATION

A process in which platelets stick together and stick to artery walls; a part of blood clotting.

POLYUNSATURATED FAT

The predominant fat in common vegetable oils such as

corn, safflower, sunflower, cottonseed, soybean and
walnut oils.

PROGESTERONE
A female hormone; hormone-replacement therapy
(HRT) containing progesterone appears to raise triglyc-
erides less significantly than therapies which do not.

RELATIVE RISK
A comparison of the risks between two different groups.

SATURATED FATS
Cholesterol-raising fats, hard at room temperature, such
as butter and lard.

SEROTONIN
A brain neurotransmitter which helps to inhibit impulsive
behaviour. In some animal studies, low cholesterol levels
have been linked with low levels of serotonin.

SIMVASTATIN
A cholesterol-lowering drug which interferes with the
body's ability to make cholesterol in the liver; an **HMG
CoA reductase inhibitor**.

STEARIC ACID
A component of the saturated fats found in red meat
and chocolate, thought not to raise LDL cholesterol
levels.

GLOSSARY

STEROLS
The class of compounds to which cholesterol belongs.

TRANS FATTY ACIDS
Compounds found in hydrogenated fats which have the same cholesterol-raising properties as saturated fats.

TRIGLYCERIDES
Fatty compounds found in the blood which contain three chains of fatty acids linked to one glycerol (glycerine) molecule.

VASOSPASMS
Contractions of the blood vessels.

VERY LOW-DENSITY LIPOPROTEIN (VLDL)
A type of lipoprotein converted in the body to LDL cholesterol and triglycerides. Most forms of VLDL do not appear to play a role in the development of atherosclerosis.

XANTHOMAS
Fatty deposits of cholesterol in the tendons, associated with inherited cholesterol disorders.

SELECTED BIBLIOGRAPHY

'Blood cholesterol and brain cancer', *British Medical Journal* 11 February 1995: 367

'Blood cholesterol: lipid measurement value', *Journal of the American Medical Association* March 25 1992: 1649

'Blood cholesterol: lowering', *British Medical Journal* 17 June 1989: 1594

'Blood cholesterol measurement', *British Journal of Hospital Medicine* 6 May 1992: 639

'Childhood cholesterol screening', *Journal of the American Medical Association* June 12 1991: 3003

'Childhood cholesterol screening', *Journal of the American Medical Association* January 1 1992: 100

'Children and cholesterol fat streaks – LDL HDL', *Journal of the American Medical Association* February 5 1992

'Cholesterol', *British Medical Journal* 5 February 1994: 351

'Cholesterol and aggression', *Lancet* 24 October 1992: 995

'Cholesterol blood measurement', *Pulse* 98 (1992)

'Cholesterol and CHD coronary thrombosis', *Journal of the American Medical Association* December 19 1990

'Cholesterol and coronary heart disease', *Journal of the American Medical Association* February 12 1992: 816

'Cholesterol and coronary heart disease', *British Medical Journal* 4 July 1992: 15

'Cholesterol crystal emboli', *Lancet* 15 June 1996: 1641

'Cholesterol dangers', *British Medical Journal* 22 May 1993: 1355 1367

'Cholesterol and depression', *Lancet* 9 January 1993: 75

'Cholesterol and depression', *British Medical Journal* 11 January 1997: 143

'Cholesterol, diastolic BP and stroke', *Lancet* 23 December 1995: 1647

'Cholesterol and eggs', *Journal of the American Medical Association* September 4 1991: 1192

'Cholesterol embolism', *Lancet* 30 November 1991: 1365

'Cholesterol facts', *Journal of the American Medical Association* December 19 1990: 3078

'Cholesterol, fibre and bile acids', *Lancet* 17 February 1996: 415

'Cholesterol and heart disease', *New England Journal of Medicine* 4 February 1993: 313

'Cholesterol and heart disease', *Journal of the Royal Society of Medicine* August 1994: 450

'Cholesterol and heart disease Doll', *New Scientist* 21 November 1992: 32

'Cholesterol: is intervention worth while?' *British Medical Journal* 11 May 1991: 1119

'Cholesterol levels soaring in Japan', *New Scientist* 2 September 1995: 5

'Cholesterol levels and suicide', *British Medical Journal* 24 June 1995: 1632

'Cholesterol levels – when to intervene', *Pulse* 28

'Cholesterol-lowering and coronary heart disease', *Lancet* 2 December 1995: 1467

'Cholesterol-lowering does not reduce atherosclerosis', *Lancet* 29 October 1994: 1182

'Cholesterol-lowering drugs', *British Medical Journal* 15 February 1992: 431

'Cholesterol-lowering and heart disease', *British Medical Journal* 15 May 1993: 1313

'Cholesterol and margarine', *Scientific American* January 1991: 14

'Cholesterol – papers' comments', *British Medical Journal* 16 April 1994: 1025

'Cholesterol and older people', *British Journal of Hospital Medicine* November 1991: 323

'Cholesterol screening', *British Medical Journal* 17 June 1989: 1593

'Cholesterol screening', *British Medical Journal* 2 September 1989: 606

'Cholesterol screening', *British Medical Journal* 22 September 1990: 584

'Cholesterol and Sitostanol-ester margarine', *New England Journal of Medicine* November 16 1995: 1308

'Cholesterol and survival', *Lancet* 20 May 1995: 1274

'Cholesterol and violence', *British Journal of Hospital Medicine* 6 April 1994: 329

'Cholesterol and violent death', *British Medical Journal* 13 August 1994: 421

'Cholesterol and violent death', *British Medical Journal* 5
   November 1994: 1228

'Cholesterol is vital for life', *New Scientist* 19 October
   1996: 18

'Cholesterol: the whole story', *Journal of the American
   Medical Association* December 19 1990

'Coffee beans and cholesterol-raising factor', *Journal of
   the Royal Society of Medicine* November 1996: 618

'Coffee and blood lipids cholesterol', *Journal of the Royal
   Society of Medicine* 3 September 1994: 506

'Coffee and cholesterol', *British Medical Journal* 29
   October 1988: 1103

'Coffee and cholesterol', *New England Journal of
   Medicine* November 23 1989: 1432

'Coffee and cholesterol', *Journal of the American Medical
   Association* February 12 1992: 811

'Coffee, cholesterol, heart disease', *British Medical Journal*
   6 April 1991: 804

'Cooking oil and blood cholesterol levels', *British Medical
   Journal* 26 October 1996: 1044

'Coronary deaths: familial hypercholesterolaemia', *British
   Medical Journal* 12 October 1991

'Coronary heart disease and cholesterol in the elderly',
   British Medical Journal 13 July 1991: 69

'Coronary heart disease: populations, low cholesterol',
   British Medical Journal 3 August 1991

'Dietary serum cholesterol', *British Medical Journal* 19
   October 1991: 953

'Eating less fat cholesterol and mortality', *Journal of the
   American Medical Association* June 26 1991

'Estimating true cholesterol level', *Journal of the American Medical Association* September 25 1991: 1678

'Exercise increases good diet drops in cholesterol', *Lancet* 23 March 1996: 819

'Fibre in oats and cholesterol', *Journal of the American Medical Association* April 10 1991: 1833

'HDL cholesterol, alcohol and heart disease', *British Medical Journal* 11 May 1996: 1200

'HDL cholesterol and heart attacks in female runners', *New England Journal of Medicine* May 16 1996: 1298

'High blood cholesterol', *Journal of the American Medical Association* March 3 1993: 1133

'High blood cholesterol risks simvastatin', *British Medical Journal* 20 May 1995: 1280

'Home cholesterol testing', *Lancet* 5 December 1992: 1386

'Hypercholesterolaemia, asymptomatic', *British Medical Journal* 16 March 1991: 605

'Low cholesterol and depression', *British Medical Journal* 21 May 1994: 1328

'Low cholesterol depression', *New Scientist* 29 April 1995: 10

'Low cholesterol and suicide', *Lancet* 21 March 1992: 727

'Lowered cholesterol and mood disturbance disproved', *British Medical Journal* 13 July 1996: 75

'McDonalds and cholesterol', *Journal of the American Medical Association* December 19 1990: 3071

'Pig liver transplant cells keep cholesterol at bay', *New Scientist* 18 January 1997: 19

'Plasma cholesterol and saturated fat intake', *British Medical Journal* 11 November 1995: 1260

'Serum cholesterol', *Journal of the American Medical Association* June 16 1993: 3002

'Serum cholesterol and low mood', *British Medical Journal* 14 September 1996: 637

'Serum cholesterol and mortality', *British Medical Journal* 12 August 1995: 409

'Soy proteins and blood lipids cholesterol', *New England Journal of Medicine* August 3 1995: 276

'Total cholesterol concentration and mortality', *British Medical Journal* 23 September 1995: 779

INDEX